THE
MEDiTERRANEAN
DIET COOKBOOK
FOR BEGINNERS

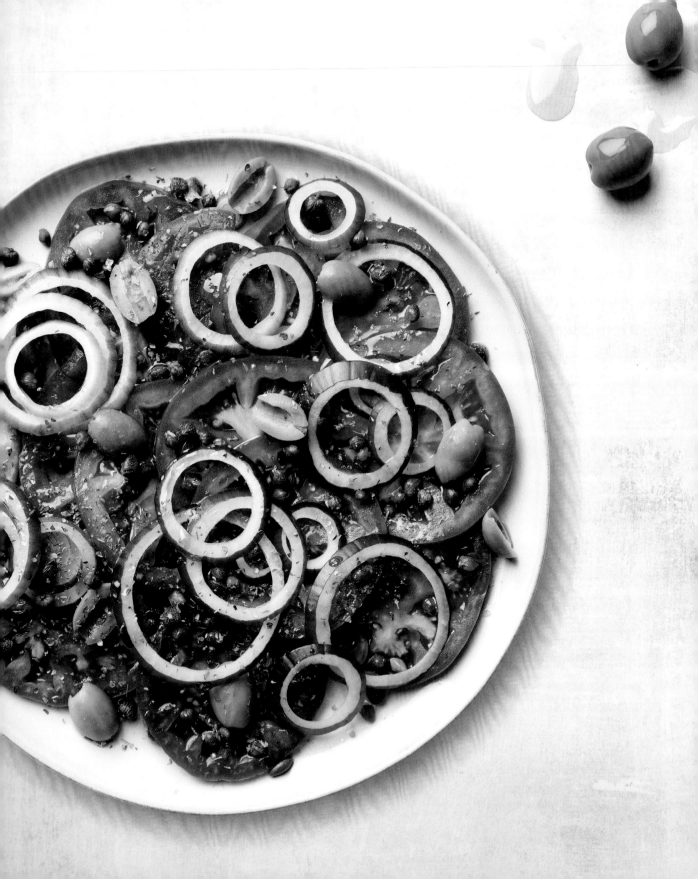

THE MEDITERRANEAN DIET COOKBOOK FOR BEGINNERS

Meal plans, expert guidance, & 100 recipes to get you started

ELENA PARAVANTES, RDN of OliveTomato.com

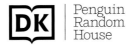

Publisher Mike Sanders
Senior Editor Brook Farling
Senior Designer Jessica Lee
Art Director William Thomas
Photographer Daniel Showalter
Food Stylist Lovoni Walker
Proofreader Georgette Beatty
Indexer Celia McCoy

First American Edition, 2020
Published in the United States by DK Publishing
1745 Broadway, 20th Floor, New York, NY 10019

The authorized representative in the EEA is Dorling Kindersley Verlag
GmbH. Arnulfstr. 124, 80636 Munich, Germany

Copyright © 2020 Elena Paravantes
24 25 16 15 14
017-318453-DEC2020

Library of Congress Catalog Number: 2020930828
ISBN: 978-1-4654-9767-3

DK books are available at special discounts when purchased in bulk for
sales promotions, premiums, fund-raising, or educational use. For
details, contact
SpecialSales@dk.com

Author photo on page 5 © Elena Paravantes
All other images © Dorling Kindersley Limited

Printed and bound in China

For the curious
www.dk.com

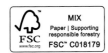

MIX
Paper | Supporting
responsible forestry
FSC™ C018179

This book was made with Forest
Stewardship Council ™ certified
paper - one small step in DK's
commitment to a sustainable future.
For more information go to
www.dk.com/our-green-pledge

ABOUT THE AUTHOR

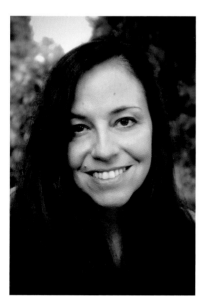

Elena Paravantes, RDN, is the creator of olivetomato.com, the top online resource for the authentic Mediterranean diet. She is a registered dietitian nutritionist, writer, consultant, and lecturer with more than 20 years of professional experience both in the United States and Greece. An award-winning expert on the Greek Mediterranean diet, her interviews and articles have appeared in publications and websites, including *U.S. News & World Report,* CNN, *Prevention, Men's Health, Women's Health, Shape, Fitness, Parade,* Salon, *Today's Dietitian, Food & Nutrition,* and NPR. She is the past food and nutrition editor of the Greek editions of *Men's Health* and *Prevention* magazines. Elena is frequently invited to speak about issues related to the Mediterranean diet and olive oil for international and national conferences and has collaborated with a number of institutions, including Yale University, Loyola University, the University of Missouri, Louisiana State University, American College of Greece, and American University of Madaba in Jordan.

ACKNOWLEDGMENTS

First and foremost, I would like to thank my publishers and the team at DK/Alpha Books for producing a book that means so much to me.

A huge thank you to my editor, Brook Farling, who supported my approach from start to finish, guided me through the process, and transformed my vision into a valuable book.

I also want to thank my readers for requesting and gently pushing me to put my recipes and guidance in a book.

A very special thank you goes to my husband, Patrick, who has been encouraging me to write a book for years and believing in the importance of my cause. And to our two little boys, who have been my fearless and adventurous recipe critics.

Finally, I am eternally grateful to my parents for being the inspiration for my work and raising me to savor, appreciate, and cherish our beloved Mediterranean diet.

CONTENTS

6: SALADS

7: SNACKS AND APPETIZERS

8: DESSERTS

FOREWORD

The Mediterranean diet is a traditional eating pattern that encompasses identified traditional foods. When the Mediterranean diet was acknowledged by the United Nations body, UNESCO, as an intangible cultural heritage, the definition was established as a set of skills, knowledge, practices, and traditions ranging from the landscape to the table, including the crops, harvesting, fishing, conservation, processing, preparation and, in particular, consumption of food. These traditions and traditional foods are the cornerstones for this recognized healthy diet pattern.

In recent years, several myths and misconceptions associated with the traditional Mediterranean diet have emerged and should be clearly addressed and dispelled, particularly those that label as "Mediterranean" eating patterns that are not in line with the traditional diet.

The Mediterranean Diet Cookbook for Beginners provides valuable information on the traditional Mediterranean diet and its representative foods, identifying mainly Greek foods, most of which are virtually unknown, together with some recipes from southern Italy. Indeed, this is a much-needed book in this time of confusion.

Ms. Paravantes provides us with an informed approach to the traditional Mediterranean diet, offering a clear method to introduce this dietary pattern with its health benefits, delicious taste, and contribution as a sustainable food system.

Antonia Trichopoulou, M.D.
President, Hellenic Health Foundation
Professor Emeritus, National and Kapodistrian University of Athens Medical School

INTRODUCTION

What if I told you that there is a diet that is delicious, doesn't leave you hungry, and still keeps you thin and healthy? There is, and the secret is that it's not really a diet.

Enter the Mediterranean diet, a traditional eating pattern that was virtually unknown until recently, but has now become the gold standard of healthy diets. Hundreds of scientific studies support its numerous health benefits, and it's no wonder that it's become so popular—it's delicious! And the best part is, once you adopt the Mediterranean diet lifestyle, you won't even feel like you're on a diet—it's a healthier way of eating that you can follow for a lifetime.

With all of the proven science behind the Mediterranean diet, however, there is still a great deal of confusion about this eating pattern. If you don't know where to start, you are not alone. Despite its popularity, much of the available information on the Mediterranean diet is inconsistent, inaccurate, and often limited to vague and stereotypical descriptions of eating a lot of fish and drinking copious amounts of wine. Quite often you might see versions of the Mediterranean diet that resemble a typical westernized weight loss diet. These versions do not represent a true Mediterranean diet, but adulterated versions that will have little to no positive impact on your health. And I should know! Being a Greek American nutritionist and registered dietitian, I was raised on the Mediterranean diet both in Greece and the United States, and I have firsthand knowledge of the diet and years of experience with this way of eating.

As a nutritionist, I counsel my patients on the real Mediterranean diet. And as a longtime magazine writer and editor, I have always made sure that the Mediterranean diet is portrayed correctly in my writing. When I wanted to reach an even larger audience, I started my own website dedicated only to the Mediterranean diet, naming it olivetomato.com (two basic ingredients of Mediterranean cuisine). And now, with this book, I am taking it a step further by sharing my Mediterranean diet knowledge, meal plans, recipes, and guidelines that are based on my personal experience with the diet and extensive research and interviews with top researchers and Mediterranean residents and elders who follow the diet—all to create simple yet authentic recipes and lifestyle practices that will have a truly positive impact on your health.

With *The Mediterranean Diet Cookbook for Beginners*, you'll experience the real Mediterranean diet. I provide a lifetime of experience along with tried-and-true family recipes—and some new ones—that are all made using accessible ingredients. This book also offers a set of easy-to-follow core guidelines that are based on the traditional Mediterranean way of eating, elaborating on key concepts of the true Mediterranean lifestyle that can lead to improved health and more enjoyment of the food you eat. I've included all the tools you need to get started, including cooking tips, a lifestyle guide, a shopping list, meal descriptions, and a detailed 2-week meal plan. It really is that easy!

You know that the Mediterranean diet is good for you, and now you can follow it from any part of the world, do it the right way, and gain all the health benefits of this revolutionary way of eating and living.

—Elena Paravantes

CHAPTER ONE
INTRODUCTION

WHAT IS THE *AUTHENTiC* MEDiTERRANEAN DIET?

The authentic Mediterranean diet is a well-established eating and lifestyle pattern among populations in certain areas of the Mediterranean that is associated with longevity and numerous other health benefits. The diet features a high intake of vegetable dishes, often consumed as main courses, and a generous use of extra virgin olive oil, particularly in vegetable dishes, while meat intake is limited to only a few servings each month. But it's not only about food. The Mediterranean diet also is a way of life based on positive social connections, life enjoyment, self-care, productivity, and regular physical activity.

THE ORIGINS OF THE DIET

In antiquity, a Mediterranean diet model existed as the Mediterranean triad: wheat (bread), grapevines (wine), and olive trees (olive oil). The first known modern study of the Mediterranean diet occurred somewhat accidentally in 1948. The Greek government had invited the Rockefeller Foundation to research the post-war standard of living on the Greek island of Crete. During its research, the foundation discovered that the eating habits of the people living in rural Crete were nutritionally comparable to the U.S. standards of the time. This was surprising because the diet included almost no meat, and instead consisted mainly of wild greens, beans, vegetables, fruits, bread, homemade wine, and plenty of olive oil.

In the next few years, there was an increased interest in the eating habits found in the Mediterranean, and particularly in southern Europe. In the 1950s, U.S. physiologist Ancel Keys noticed that American businessmen who followed a meat and potatoes–type diet—which was considered balanced in the United States at the time—had higher rates of cardiovascular

disease compared to southern European men who followed a plant-based diet. The European men were much healthier than the American men, even though their diets were quite limited, according to U.S. nutrition standards. This led Keys to his famous Seven Countries Study, which showed that a plant-based diet rich in good fats, such as olive oil, but with little meat, was associated with better health and increased longevity, particularly on the Greek island of Crete, where, at the time, Cretan men had the highest life expectancy in the world. This discovery paved the way for more research in Mediterranean countries such as Greece and Italy.

In 1993, a model of the Mediterranean diet, in the form of a preliminary food pyramid based on the Cretan diet, was presented at a conference organized by the Harvard School of Public Health and Oldways, a nonprofit nutrition organization. A year later, the same researchers published an article describing the Mediterranean diet, and noted that the Mediterranean diet pyramid was based on food patterns typical of Crete, much of the rest of Greece, and southern Italy in the early 1960s.

It's because of this early research that the Mediterranean diet has garnered significant attention today from both the public and culinary professionals, and is now considered the gold standard of diets by the scientific community.

It's important to note that the authentic Mediterranean diet (which is what this book is based on) is followed only in certain areas of the Mediterranean. This diet does not reflect the eating patterns of the entire Mediterranean region—some Mediterranean countries use very little olive oil, while in others meat is consumed quite often. Only certain areas of the Mediterranean, including the island of Crete, most of Greece, and the southern region of Italy, follow the specific eating patterns that are associated with these significant health benefits. And while all regions of the Mediterranean feature wonderful dishes that might fit into a Mediterranean diet, the eating pattern for the authentic Mediterranean diet is very specific and isolated to these regions.

WHAT SETS THE AUTHENTIC MEDITERRANEAN DIET APART?

What makes this diet different than other "healthy" diets? First of all, it's not really a diet, and it's certainly not a plan that will make you feel deprived. This way of eating and living has evolved naturally in specific areas of the Mediterranean region, and has been followed and enjoyed for generations. It's an ideal way of eating because it's realistic and it also tastes good. Additionally, it is, by far, one of the most researched diets in existence and also the one with the most wide-ranging benefits. Finally, the Mediterranean diet is considered ideal not only because of its health benefits and palatability, but also because of its environmental sustainability. This is a diet that is both good for you and good for the planet.

THE HEALTH BENEFITS OF THE MEDITERRANEAN DIET

The Mediterranean diet is the most extensively studied diet in the world. The research is abundant and ongoing, with more scientific evidence supporting its benefits compared to any other diet—and those benefits are significant.

IT PROTECTS THE HEART

The Mediterranean diet protects the body from heart disease in a number of ways: it lowers bad cholesterol levels, it controls blood pressure, and it lowers the risk of obesity, including the development of abdominal fat. A comprehensive body of evidence supports the Mediterranean diet as a heart-healthy diet, even when compared to conventional low-fat diets. Research has shown that adherence to a Mediterranean diet is associated with up to a 25 percent reduced risk of developing cardiovascular disease, and it's shown to have a protective benefit for individuals who already have heart disease. A study by Greek researchers published in the *Archives of Internal Medicine* showed that individuals with coronary artery disease had a 27 percent lower risk of mortality when they followed the Mediterranean diet. Other studies have pointed out that the Mediterranean diet can have the same potential benefits as medication when it comes to treating heart disease. Another study, the EPIC-Norfolk, found that the Mediterranean diet was associated with lower heart disease incidence and mortality in a non-Mediterranean population.

IT PROTECTS FROM DIABETES

Some people believe that the Mediterranean diet is a high-carbohydrate diet and inappropriate for individuals with diabetes, but that's simply not the case. In truth, it's a moderate-carbohydrate diet that has been shown to protect against the oxidative stress and inflammation that can lead to chronic diseases such as diabetes. Scientific reviews have shown that following the Mediterranean diet can reduce the risk of diabetes by up to 50 percent. Other studies have shown that individuals with diabetes who follow the Mediterranean diet have experienced improved blood sugar control and maintained a healthier weight. Another study showed that newly diagnosed individuals may be able to delay taking diabetes medication by following the Mediterranean diet.

IT CAN PROTECT FROM CERTAIN TYPES OF CANCER

Due to its abundance of antioxidants, omega-3 fatty acids, and fiber, the Mediterranean diet can help protect against certain types of cancer by modifying hormones and other factors related to cancer development. The nutrients in the diet can help reduce inflammation, avoid damage to DNA, and prevent metastasis, which is the spread of cancer cells. Research has shown that those following the Mediterranean diet have a reduced risk of overall cancer mortality, with protection from a number of cancers, including breast, prostate, colorectal, and upper respiratory tract cancers.

IT CAN KEEP YOUR BRAIN SHARP

The past decade has seen an increased interest in how the Mediterranean diet affects cognitive function, the mental process that allows us to carry out tasks. Studies have shown that the Mediterranean diet is associated with less mental decline and dementia and a reduced risk of developing Alzheimer's disease by up to 40 percent. A French study showed that the Mediterranean diet can potentially delay cognitive decline by up to 10 years. Several studies have also found improvement in memory and problem-solving skills in those who follow the diet.

IT WILL HELP YOU LOSE WEIGHT AND MAINTAIN A HEALTHY WEIGHT

The same qualities of the Mediterranean diet that help protect from heart disease also help practitioners maintain a normal weight and reduce waistline fat. A European study with more than 490,000 participants showed that the Mediterranean diet was associated with reduced abdominal fat. Another study in the United States with more than 10,000 participants found that those following the Mediterranean diet in middle age experienced less age-related weight gain. Numerous other studies have compared the Mediterranean diet to more restrictive diets and found that the Mediterranean style of eating resulted in long-term weight loss, long-term adherence to the diet, and a reduction in blood pressure and blood sugar levels.

IT CAN IMPROVE YOUR MOOD

An overview of more than 40 studies found a strong association between the Mediterranean diet and a reduced risk of depression. A westernized diet can cause damage to the brain through oxidative stress, but the Mediterranean diet, rich in antioxidants, can help protect the brain and reduce damage. Another study from Australia found that the Mediterranean diet can improve mood in individuals who suffer from depression by up to 30 percent. A Greek study found that adherence to the Mediterranean diet was associated with a decreased likelihood of developing symptoms of depression later in life.

IT CAN HELP YOU LIVE LONGER— AND BETTER

Researchers first noted in the 1950s and 1960s that individuals in certain parts of the Mediterranean had higher life expectancies compared to people in other parts of the world. Today, larger studies have proven that the Mediterranean diet is, in fact, associated with longer life expectancies, and individuals following the Mediterranean diet are more likely to live longer. Following the Mediterranean diet also improves quality of life and well-being, and equates to less frailty and disability in old age. It's not enough to just live long; it's important to live well.

ADDITIONAL BENEFITS

Researchers are still studying numerous other health conditions that the Mediterranean diet may have a positive impact on, including Parkinson's disease, arthritis, eye health, dental health, fertility health, lung issues, and more. We do already know it benefits the gut microbiome—a group of microorganisms present in the gastrointestinal tract that can help protect against chronic disease.

THE PRINCIPLES OF AN AUTHENTIC MEDITERRANEAN DIET

You may already be familiar with some of the general guidelines and philosophies of the Mediterranean diet, while others you may be surprised to learn, but one thing is for certain: once you fully understand the principles of this incredibly healthy eating pattern, it will become second nature to you.

KEY PRINCIPLES OF THE MEDITERRANEAN DIET

The authentic Mediterranean diet is based on these key principles:

- **The main ingredients are plants.** Most of your food will come from plant sources, particularly vegetables, and the basis of your diet will be vegetables and beans. Other plant foods that will supplement your diet include fruits, nuts, and seeds.

- **There is an emphasis on fresh and minimally processed foods.** The Mediterranean diet generally does not include many prepackaged or processed foods. And although some minimally processed foods, such as bread and frozen vegetables, will still be a part of your diet, highly processed foods such as chips or rice mixes will not be, even if they say "Mediterranean" on the packaging.

- **Local and seasonal ingredients are preferred.** This means that you should look for vegetables that are in season where you live. Eating with the seasons is recommended because it provides variety in your diet throughout the year, and variety can have an additional protective impact on your health.

- **Cooking methods and dishes are based on simple, clean flavors and straightforward preparations.** Home cooking should be simple with easy-to-find ingredients.

- **Extra virgin olive oil is the main source of fat.** Other oils are not used. Extra virgin olive oil is used exclusively for all roasting, frying, and sautéing.

- **Dairy products, particularly cheese, are protein supplements and accompany vegetable-based foods.** Almost all vegetable dishes in the Mediterranean diet are accompanied by cheese.

- **Fish and poultry are consumed in moderation and not every day.** Fatty fish like sardines, anchovies, mackerel, and salmon are preferable due to their high omega-3 fatty acid content.

- **Desserts are consumed only on special occasions.** A bit of sugar in your coffee or honey in tea or yogurt is fine, but as a general rule, sweets should be enjoyed only in moderation.

- **Beverages are mainly water, wine (with food), coffee, tea, and herbal beverages.** Juices, smoothies, and soft drinks generally are not consumed on a daily basis, and instead should be consumed only on special occasions.

- **Red meat, including pork, is consumed as a main course about once a week.** Red meat can also be used in small amounts to "season" vegetable dishes, but it should not be consumed in large quantities or on a regular basis.

MEDITERRANEAN DIET MACRONUTRIENTS

Macronutrients—or *macros*—refers to the three primary nutrients your body uses in large amounts: carbohydrates, fats, and protein. Analysis of the Mediterranean diet has revealed a very specific ratio of these nutrients that should be consumed for optimum benefit.

CARBOHYDRATES
(40–45% of daily caloric intake)
Research has shown that a carbohydrate intake ranging from 40 to 50% is ideal for health and longevity and is associated with lower mortality rates. Contrary to what many people believe, the Mediterranean diet is not a high-carbohydrate diet. The authentic Mediterranean diet is not about eating large quantities of pasta, pizza, and bread, but instead is about consuming a high volume of vegetables, olive oil, and healthy plant proteins. Because most main meals on the diet are vegetable-based, your carbohydrates will come from accompaniments such as bread or rice. A dish made mainly from carbohydrates, such as pasta, is typically consumed no more than twice a week.

FAT
(35–40% of daily caloric intake)
The dietary fat in the Mediterranean diet is considered moderate. It was once thought that any healthy diet had to be low-fat, but we now know that a moderate-fat diet can be good both for the heart and for weight loss. Remember those Cretan men in the 1960s? They consumed large amounts of olive oil and had extremely low rates of heart disease. What's important is not the amount of fat that is consumed, but rather the type of fat consumed. The fat in the Mediterranean diet comes mostly from extra virgin olive oil, which is mainly an unsaturated fat rich in antioxidants. Other sources of healthy fats in the diet include fatty fish, walnuts, and some types of greens, all of which contain highly beneficial omega-3 fatty acids. It's important not to try to follow a low-fat Mediterranean diet because a true Mediterranean diet can never be low-fat. All those good fats have proven health benefits, provide satiety and flavor, and best of all, make eating large amounts of vegetables both easy and enjoyable.

PROTEIN
(20% of daily caloric intake)
Even though the Mediterranean diet is not a meat-rich diet, protein intake on the diet is more than adequate. The main sources of protein are beans, eggs, yogurt, cheese, poultry, fatty fish, and nuts. Plant-based sources of protein also provide fiber and antioxidants.

A NOTE BEFORE TRANSITIONING TO THE MEDITERRANEAN DIET

Before starting this diet, you should consult with your physician to ensure that switching to the Mediterranean diet is the optimal choice for your health. The information contained in this book is not meant to be used to diagnose or treat any specific medical condition, nor is it intended as a substitute for medical advice or treatment from a medical doctor.

THE MEDITERRANEAN DIET—FREQUENTLY ASKED QUESTIONS

It can be confusing to know if the Mediterranean is appropriate for you and your health—and there is plenty of misinformation out there regarding the diet. Because so much misinformation exists, here are some answers to some of the most frequently asked questions I receive.

CAN I LOSE WEIGHT ON THIS DIET?

Yes! Research has shown that the Mediterranean diet can result in equal or greater weight loss compared to low-fat and low-carbohydrate diets. Studies have also shown that the Mediterranean diet is associated with lower body fat and is the best diet for keeping weight off. The secret of following the Mediterranean diet for weight loss, particularly for the long term, is that it's not really a "diet," so you won't feel deprived like you might on a more restrictive diet. This means you can eat this way for a lifetime, and you'll get the added benefit of protection from many chronic diseases and conditions. With that said, there are certain key principles of the diet to keep in mind that play an important role in weight control: eating your main meal earlier in the day, consuming mostly vegetables, avoiding processed foods (particularly starches), and drinking mostly water and herbal beverages.

HOW DO I REDUCE MEAT INTAKE?

If you are accustomed to eating meat almost every day, don't worry! You still will be eating some meat, but it will be consumed differently, and in smaller amounts. Here are some general guidelines for how to reduce your meat intake:

- Begin by gradually eating less meat every day, reducing it little by little and replacing it with more hearty vegetables.
- Consume meat as a side, not as the centerpiece of the meal.
- Eat fatty fish, which is richer in flavor and can provide satiety, in place of meat.
- Remove deli meats from sandwiches, and instead use your favorite cheese with vegetables and nut butters to create a hearty sandwich.
- Don't replace meat with carbohydrates. Instead make sure you are eating enough good fats to keep you full and satisfied.

CAN I FOLLOW THIS DIET IF I AM VEGAN?

You can. A little-known fact about the Mediterranean diet is that the traditional Greek diet, which was used as a model for the Mediterranean diet, was vegan for almost half the year due to religious practices. Meat plays a secondary role in the diet, and as a result, the cuisine features numerous vegan options, including hearty vegetables dishes, a variety of bean recipes like casseroles, and vegetable patties and dips, all making it an ideal eating pattern for vegans. Vegans can also supplement the diet with grains, nuts (particularly walnuts), and seed and nut butters.

ARE THERE GLUTEN-FREE OPTIONS?

Absolutely. Because the majority of dishes are vegetable-based, there are numerous choices for those wishing to avoid gluten. With the exception of some pasta dishes and some savory pies, most Mediterranean dishes are gluten-free. Additionally, research has shown that individuals with celiac disease who normally followed a gluten-free diet were able to improve their nutritional health without gaining weight after they switched to the Mediterranean diet.

I'M DIABETIC. SHOULD I FOLLOW A MEDITERRANEAN DIET?

Yes, you should. The Mediterranean diet, although known more for being heart-healthy, is an excellent diet for individuals with diabetes. Numerous studies have found the Mediterranean diet is associated with weight loss, reduction of blood sugar, and a delayed requirement for diabetes medications when compared to other diets. It's a moderate- to low-carb diet, based mostly on vegetables, good fats, and whole grains, and that all can result in stabilizing blood sugar levels. In addition, it's rich in antioxidants and can play an important role in the prevention and management of diabetes.

DO I HAVE TO DRINK ALCOHOL?

Absolutely not. If you do not drink alcohol, there is no reason to start now. If you do drink, know that drinking small to moderate amounts of red wine with food has been associated with certain health benefits and is a part of the traditional Mediterranean diet. If you prefer not to drink, you'll still get the same tremendous benefits of this diet even if you choose not to consume alcohol.

WHAT SHOULD I EAT WHEN I'M OUT?

Many restaurant offerings are consistent with the Mediterranean diet principles:

- For breakfast, choose eggs simply prepared along with a side of fresh fruit. You can also choose yogurt with fresh fruit. Avoid dishes with numerous ingredients and complex preparations.
- For lunch, if you are going to choose a sandwich, skip the meat, choose whole-grain bread, and fill the sandwich with cheese, healthy spreads such as hummus, tapenade, tahini, or almond butter, and plenty of vegetables.
- If you choose a salad, top it with cheese and nuts. If you add chicken, choose grilled options. And don't forget to use olive oil for your dressing!
- For dinner, basic options can include grilled fish or sautéed shrimp on a bed of vegetables. And in the spirit of the Mediterranean diet, if you are out for a special occasion, have some dessert!

IS THIS DIET FOR THE WHOLE FAMILY?

It is. In fact, studies have shown that children who follow a Mediterranean diet are more likely to maintain a normal weight, and the same goes for pregnant women. Vegetables cooked the traditional Mediterranean diet way are so flavorful and palatable, even the pickiest of adults and children will enjoy them

KID-FRIENDLY MEDITERRANEAN DIET SUBSTITUTIONS

- Where butter is used in some recipes, such as grilled cheese sandwiches, use olive oil instead.
- Use hummus or olive tapenade in place of a ranch dip for vegetables.
- Instead of chips, serve olives with whole-wheat breadsticks.
- Replace high-sodium snacks with fresh mozzarella balls served with cherry tomatoes.
- In place of sugary snacks, substitute a trail mix made with raisins, walnuts, and almonds.

THE MEDiTERRANEAN LiFESTYLE

Some key aspects of the Mediterranean diet go beyond what you eat. These lifestyle practices are characteristic of populations in the Mediterranean and play an important role in the longevity seen in this region. Although they are not necessarily food-related, they can have a positive impact on your overall health and well-being.

SOCIALIZING INFORMALLY

One of the key aspects of a Mediterranean lifestyle is the social factor. By this I mean the simple act of communicating with the ones around you, and for no particular reason other than to stay connected. Saying hello to neighbors, asking how the cashier at your local grocery store is doing, or calling a friend just to talk are examples of what I call unplanned or informal socializing. These actions can help keep you connected to the world and also provide a sense of wellness.

EATING WITH COMPANY

The ancient Greeks strove to achieve what they called a civilized lifestyle, and one of the ways they did this was to socialize while eating. In the Mediterranean, eating is not an act of merely satisfying the physical need of hunger, but rather a communal event. Conviviality, meaning to eat and drink in good company, is an important aspect of the Mediterranean diet, and there are several small habits you can adopt to practice this principle. At work, you can take a break and make an effort to eat with coworkers. At home, dinner is an opportunity to eat and stay connected with family members. When going out for a meal, consider it an opportunity to not only eat good food but also to discuss, laugh, and relax with the people you enjoy being around most.

BEING ACTIVE

The idea of physical activity within a Mediterranean diet is about a state of mind, and not just about spending an hour in the gym. It means walking as often as possible, doing housework and gardening, walking to your local store, taking the stairs, or parking far away from a building to get in those extra steps. These small habits all can lead to a more active lifestyle that goes beyond gym time.

ENJOYING QUIET TIME

A common characteristic in many Mediterranean countries is the concept of quiet time. In Greece, it's called *mesimeri*, in Italy *riposo*, and in Spain *siesta*. It is a time to relax—usually after lunch—and take a break from what you are doing and, if you are lucky, even take a nap. It's common for many stores in these areas of the world to close during this time, and some laws even prohibit excessive noise during these periods of rest. Research has shown that a short nap can reduce blood pressure as well as lower the risk of stroke. Nowadays in larger Mediterranean cities, it is not always possible to take this midday break, although this practice is still very much alive and well in smaller communities and is common during weekends and vacations. We can all add some quiet time in our days; it refreshes our minds and bodies. If a nap is not possible, get a bit of quiet time by stepping away from the computer, closing the shades, and relaxing in your favorite chair or on the couch. You can read a book or a magazine to relax, even if it's just for 10 minutes.

HAVING A PURPOSE

Having a purpose can be something as simple as staying active each day. It can be work-related, or it can be related to little things in your life like home, garden, or cooking. It can be related to volunteering in your community or helping other people. Having a purpose can make you feel useful and productive.

BEING HOSPITABLE

The practice of welcoming guests and strangers into your home is a practice alive and well in the Mediterranean. It traces back to ancient Greece and is known as *philoxenia*, which literally translates to "friend to a stranger." Opening your home to guests offers an opportunity to socialize, connect, or help someone in need and is a reflection of who you are in society.

MEALTiMES ON THE MEDiTERRANEAN DIET

Traditional mealtimes on the Mediterranean diet may be a bit different than you are accustomed to, but there is a purpose to this rhythm of eating that will contribute to the overall benefit of following the Mediterranean diet lifestyle.

- **Breakfast and mid morning snack.** The first meal of the day is somewhat light, consisting mostly of savory flavors such as bread with tomatoes, olives, cheese, vegetable pies, or eggs, followed by a midmorning snack around 10 a.m., which can also be considered a late breakfast.

- **Lunch.** Lunch is the largest meal of the day and is usually consumed around 1 p.m. or as late as 4 p.m. Weekday lunches are generally vegetable-based and consumed with a small amount of starch such as bread or rice and cheese, while weekend lunches may include some meat and fish.

- **Afternoon coffee.** This practice basically signals the end of quiet time. The coffee break is around 5 p.m. and consists of coffee and a small biscuit.

- **Dinner.** Dinner is a smaller meal than lunch and can be consumed from 7 p.m. to 10 p.m. Dinner may be comprised of something quick, such as an omelet with a salad, a smaller serving of lunch, a heartier salad served on its own, or a piece of a savory pie.

What About Snacking?

Snacking per se is not a typical part of the traditional Mediterranean diet. The research is not clear on whether snacking is necessary for maintaining energy levels, but because Mediterranean meals typically are high in fiber and contain a good amount of fat, they tend to keep you feeling full for longer, making snacking generally unnecessary. However, if you are working out or your meals are spaced far apart and you find it necessary to add a snack to your diet, I suggest a piece of fruit, a handful of nuts, ½ cup of Greek yogurt, or some cherry tomatoes or other vegetables served with a bit of cheese.

WHAT To EAT AND HOW OFTEN To EAT IT

Once you transition to the Mediterranean diet, you will be eating foods from all food groups. Here is an easy-to-use guide to each group, along with information on how the foods are incorporated in the diet and how many servings you will be consuming from each food group daily.

VEGETABLES

Vegetables are at the foundation of the Mediterranean diet. Cooked or roasted vegetables typically are served as main courses and accompanied by cheese and bread. Salads may also complement meals as sides, even when the main dish is vegetable-based. Salads are abundant in the Mediterranean diet and can be eaten as main courses. Vegetables are consumed in the form of the popular Greek savory pies, patties, or dips. Using seasonal and local vegetables is always preferred, but frozen vegetables with no added ingredients are also acceptable.

Servings: at least 4 per day

Serving size: 1 cup or 2 cups salad greens

GREENS

Leafy greens are a unique component of the Cretan diet, which is considered by many to be the original Mediterranean diet. Collard greens, spinach, chard, dandelion greens, chicory, and kale are all rich in antioxidants and good sources of omega-3 fatty acids. Most commonly, they're lightly boiled and then served with olive oil and lemon, but they also can also be cooked with beans, rice, or meat.

Servings: 2–3 per week

Serving size: 2 cups (uncooked)

FRUIT

Whole local and seasonal fruits (not juice) typically are consumed after lunch and dinner. If you are including snacks in your diet, you may omit the fruit after your meal and have it as a snack instead.

Servings: 2–3 per day

Serving size: 1 medium fruit, 1 cup fresh fruit, or ¼ cup dried fruit

BEANS

Beans are a significant part of the Mediterranean diet, and all varieties are consumed. They usually are cooked and prepared with olive oil, tomato, or other vegetables and then consumed as is or with some cheese to create a complete meal. They are also served in patties and dips.

Servings: 2–3 per week

Serving size: 1 cup (cooked)

OLIVE OIL AND NUTS

Extra virgin olive oil is the main source of fat, and you will use it for cooking, baking, and sautéing. Nuts may be included in salads and some desserts or as snacks.

Servings: at least 3 and up to 6 tablespoons extra virgin olive oil per day

Serving size: 1 tablespoon olive oil or ½ ounce (14g) nuts

GRAINS AND BREAD

A slice of bread accompanies many vegetable dishes and is the most common source of carbohydrates. Savory pies are also a source; however, phyllo dough is extremely thin and does not contain many carbohydrates. It's preferable to consume whole-grain bread that does not contain any additives or preservatives. Most pasta or rice dishes are cooked with plenty of vegetables or beans.

Servings: 4–7 per day (depending on caloric level)

Serving size: 1 slice of bread, ½ cup cooked rice or pasta, or 1 medium potato

DAIRY

The main sources of dairy in the diet are cheese and yogurt. Cheeses such as feta, Parmesan, ricotta, and mizithra are consumed as accompaniments to vegetable dishes and salads. Yogurt may be eaten as is or with some nuts, honey, or fruit. Sweetened and flavored yogurts should be avoided.

Servings: 2–3 per day

Serving size: 1 cup yogurt, 1 ounce (30g) cheese

EGGS

Eggs are an important source of protein in the diet, and they're not just for breakfast. Eggs can be eaten at all times of the day and as a meal accompanied with a salad and bread.

Servings: up to 4 per week

POULTRY

Chicken is the preferred meat in the Mediterranean diet. It's typically roasted in the oven or stewed with tomatoes and herbs, and served with a salad or other vegetables.

Servings: 1–2 per week

Serving size: 6 ounces (170g)

FISH AND SEAFOOD

Fish includes mainly fatty fish like sardines, anchovies, salmon, and mackerel. Fresh options are ideal, but you can also use frozen, cured, or canned fish. Fish is typically served with stewed or boiled greens or a salad.

Servings: 2 per week

Serving size: 6 ounces (170g)

RED MEAT

Red meat, including beef, pork, and lamb, is limited on the diet and consumed either once a week in a 4- to 6-ounce (110–170g) portion or in smaller portions throughout the week. In Mediterranean cuisine, red meat is often cooked with vegetables or greens.

Servings: 1 per week

Serving size: 4–6 ounces (110–170g)

BEVERAGES

Water is the primary beverage, and at least 6 to 8 cups should be consumed each day. Teas made from herbs like chamomile, thyme, sage, and linden are also an important part of the diet and should be consumed daily. Coffee can be consumed twice per day. Alcohol is served only with meals. For those who do drink, it is recommended that men drink no more than two 5 fluid ounce (150ml) glasses of red wine daily, and women drink no more than one 5 fluid ounce (150ml) glass of red wine daily.

DESSERTS

Desserts are generally considered special occasion foods on the diet and should be enjoyed no more than once or twice per week. Honey can be used as a sweetener for herbal beverages, and sugar, in moderation, can be used in coffee.

SHOPPING FOR THE MEDITERRANEAN DIET

Transitioning to the Mediterranean diet may require making some adjustments in your shopping habits, but once you understand the philosophy of the diet, buying the right foods will come naturally.

VEGETABLES
When buying produce, focus on what is in season and grown locally. Don't feel like you have to buy a specific type of vegetable if you can't find exactly what you need; what is more important is how you prepare it. Almost any vegetable can become Mediterranean when cooked or roasted in olive oil along with herbs, onions, garlic, and tomatoes.

Buy fresh: beets, broccoli, cabbage, carrots, cauliflower, celery, cucumbers, eggplant, garlic, green beans, leeks, mushrooms, okra, onions, peas, peppers, potatoes, tomatoes, zucchini

Buy fresh or frozen: green beans, okra, peas

GREENS
Make sure to stock up on antioxidant-rich greens such as spinach, kale, collard greens, and dandelion greens. Enjoy them lightly boiled with a drizzle of olive oil.

Buy fresh: arugula, beet greens, chicory, collard greens, dandelion greens, kale, romaine lettuce, spinach, Swiss chard

Buy fresh or frozen: spinach

FRUIT
Buying seasonal fruit guarantees the best flavor. Fresh, seasonal fruit ideally is consumed whole (rather than in a smoothie or as a juice) with the skin intact, if possible.

Buy fresh: apples, apricots, avocados, cantaloupe, cherries, figs, grapefruit, grapes, lemons, mandarins, oranges, peaches, pears, tangerines, watermelon

Buy dried: apricots, dates, figs, raisins

FATS AND NUTS
Buy only high-quality extra virgin olive oil (see pages 26–27). It's preferable that any nuts be unsalted. Walnuts are ideal because they are a significant source of omega-3 fatty acids. Other sources of fat from nuts include tahini, which is sesame seed paste (choose brands that have no added sugar or other oils), and all-natural nut butters such as almond or peanut butter that contain no added sugar or oils.

What to buy: almonds, extra virgin olive oil, pine nuts, pistachios, tahini, sesame seeds, walnuts

What to avoid: vegetable and seed oils, including canola, corn, and soybean varieties

BEANS
In the Mediterranean diet, using dry beans is always preferable, but some canned varieties can be used. If you do choose to use canned beans, look for low-sodium varieties or, if using higher-sodium varieties, make sure to rinse them thoroughly to reduce the sodium content. Choose a variety of types, and keep in mind that lentils and black-eyed peas do not require soaking and can be cooked quickly. Avoid baked beans or any other preparations that may have added fat or other unwanted ingredients.

Buy dried (uncooked): black-eyed peas, butter beans, chickpeas, lentils, pinto beans, white beans

Buy canned (if needed): chickpeas, pinto beans, white beans

BREAD AND GRAINS
Look for whole-grain breads and pita breads that do not contain additives, preservatives, or fats from

unhealthy oils. Crispbreads, although not Mediterranean, can also be a good choice because they are high in fiber. For phyllo dough, which is unleavened thin sheets of dough used to make savory pies, choose brands that are low in fat.

Most pasta and rice dishes are heavy on vegetables or beans, so the fiber content is already high. For pasta, you can use regular varieties. You can also use whole-grain pasta, but the texture will be different. For rice dishes, use a medium-grain rice that provides a creamy-like texture. Avoid short-grain rice varieties because they often are too sticky, and long-grain varieties often are too dry. Brown rice can be used, but it takes longer to cook and may not have the desirable texture you're seeking. Other grains used include barley (choose hulled barley, which is whole-grain), bulgur wheat, and couscous, which should be noted is not a whole grain.

DAIRY

Choose plain Greek yogurt or yogurt made from cow's milk, sheep's milk, or goat's milk (both full-fat or low-fat varieties are acceptable). Choose yogurts that do not contain fillers, gelatin, stabilizers, protein, sweeteners, or flavorings. For cheese, choose full-fat feta, Parmesan, mozzarella, ricotta, or mizithra. Look for feta made with sheep's milk and not cow's milk.

MEATS AND POULTRY

Choose grass-fed veal, pork, ground beef, and lamb. For poultry, look for whole chickens or chicken pieces. Avoid processed meats and deli meats such as bacon, salami, bologna, and sausages.

FISH AND SEAFOOD

Choose fresh or frozen fatty fish like sardines, anchovies, mackerel, salmon, herring, and trout. Although not all of these are Mediterranean, they are all rich in omega-3 fatty acids. Other fish, such as cod, sea bass, grouper, sea bream, and whitebait, can also be added to the diet.

Buy fresh or frozen: anchovies, calamari, crab, crayfish, herring, lobster, octopus, mackerel, mussels, salmon, sardines, shrimp, trout

Buy canned: anchovies and sardines packed in olive oil, tuna packed in water

PANTRY ITEMS

Look for Greek-style processed olives, which contain the highest level of antioxidants. Capers, sun-dried tomatoes, and roasted bell peppers can be added to various recipes for a burst of flavor. Honey is the primary sweetener on the diet. Make sure it's pure honey and does not contain other ingredients. Keep a stock of chamomile, sage, linden, and Greek mountain teas on hand as well.

Frequently used pantry items: balsamic vinegar, canned crushed tomatoes, capers, honey, Kalamata olives, red wine vinegar, sugar, sun-dried tomatoes (packed in olive oil), tomato paste

Frequently used herbs and spices: allspice, basil, black pepper, cumin, dill, fine sea salt, ground cinnamon, kosher salt, mint, oregano, parsley

WHAT To AVOID WHEN SHOPPING

To make good choices when grocery shopping, ask yourself if a person living in a Mediterranean village would have the food or ingredient as a part of their diet. If the answer is "no," you probably shouldn't buy it.

Of course, there are exceptions, but in general, focus on buying whole, real foods. Avoid ultra-processed foods that contain little to no whole foods but plenty of artificial additives and preservatives shown to cause weight gain and chronic health issues.

Here are some ultra-processed foods to avoid:

- Frozen foods, including pizza, waffles, french fries, and chicken nuggets
- Sweetened cereals or bars
- Chips and other salted, starchy snacks
- Soda and fruit drinks
- Canned soups
- Cakes, cake mixes, and cookies
- Rice and pasta mixes
- Instant noodles
- Shelf-stable breads that contain preservatives

BUYING, USING, AND STORING OLIVE OIL

Extra virgin olive oil is the cornerstone of the Mediterranean diet—every meal starts with it, whether it's in the pan or on a salad, and it provides the basis of most dishes. But to receive the full benefits of olive oil, you need to know how to choose the right one and how to use it.

THE IMPORTANCE OF OLIVE OIL IN THE MEDITERRANEAN DIET

Extra virgin olive oil is a great source of good—or *monounsaturated*—fats. The olive is actually a fruit, which means that olive oil is a juice. This juice is rich in multiple healthy substances that have potent antioxidant, anti-inflammatory, and antimicrobial properties that can help protect the body from heart disease, cancer, cognitive disorders, osteoporosis, and other chronic conditions. It's believed that olive oil contains more than 400 microcomponents, the substances mostly responsible for the healthy benefits of olive oil. This high concentration of nutrients is what sets extra virgin olive oil apart from other so-called healthy oils that don't contain the same levels of potent antioxidants, and it's also why extra virgin olive oil is so critical to Mediterranean diet cuisine.

HOW MUCH OLIVE OIL SHOULD YOU CONSUME?

Most research indicates that the protective effect of extra virgin olive oil is gained with a consumption of 40–50 grams per day, which corresponds to about 3 to 4 tablespoons extra virgin olive oil per day. This generous amount of olive oil has a double function. Not only does it provide antioxidants, but it also helps increase your consumption of vegetables and provides satiety. Cooking vegetables in olive oil makes them more palatable, and the generous recommendation for daily olive oil intake means you can eat large amounts of vegetables as a main course.

Many people worry that consuming this much olive oil may cause weight gain. Quite the contrary, research has shown that olive oil is, in fact, not associated with weight gain, which has more to do with the meals you eat and dietary patterns you follow. Most recipes in the Mediterranean diet combine vegetables with generous amounts of olive oil, but with little to no starch. This results in moderate-calorie dishes and means that the overall calories you'll be consuming, even with high amounts of olive oil, will be moderate.

USING EXTRA VIRGIN OLIVE OIL FOR COOKING AND BAKING

In the Mediterranean diet, extra virgin olive oil is your main fat for cooking and is what you use for sautéing, frying, stewing, and roasting. In addition, it's added to salads, drizzled on bread and pasta, used in sauces and dressings, and can be used for baking. There's a long-standing myth that extra virgin olive oil should not be used for frying. The reason? Smoke point. Smoke point is the temperature at which a fat or oil stops shimmering and starts to smoke after being heated to a certain temperature. This "breaking point" is an indication that an oil is breaking down, and it can lead to a burnt taste. Many people believe extra virgin olive oil has too low of a smoke point to be used for frying, but extra virgin olive oil actually has a higher smoke point than many refined olive oils. It also contains the antioxidants that reduce the rate of oxidation, making it a stable and durable cooking oil. The smoke point of extra virgin olive oil ranges from about 365°F to 410°F (185°C to 210°C), and most sautéing and frying does not surpass this point. As an added benefit, studies have shown that food fried in olive oil absorbs some of the key antioxidants from the olive oil.

STORING OLIVE OIL

The main enemies of olive oil are light, oxygen, heat, and time. Therefore, you should store olive oil in a dark, airtight container, in a cool and dark space.

After a bottle of olive oil has been opened, it should be used within 6 months, so you should avoid buying very large bottles if you will not be using it within that time period.

Olive oil should be used fresh and should not be reused. Some people may want to reuse olive oil to save money, but this is not advisable because heating olive oil more than once can result in a loss of antioxidants and flavor.

How to Buy the Right Olive Oil

There are different types of olive oil, and it's important to know what you're buying, when it was made, and where it came from.

- **Choose only extra virgin olive oil.** The potent antioxidants in olive oil are only present in significant amounts in extra virgin olive oil. For this reason, it's important to use only extra virgin olive oil. Olive oil labeled with names like "pure," "regular," "refined," or "virgin" are all lower-quality olive oils that have been refined physically and chemically, or even combined with other oils.

- **Buy the freshest olive oil possible.** Look for an expiration date and, if possible, a harvest date on the label. Ideally, you want to consume olive oil within 1 year of its harvest date. Look for oils that expire 2 years from the day you buy it. Remember: olive oil is a juice, so the fresher it is, the higher the amount of antioxidants it will contain.

- **Check the origin.** Good olive oils will include the area where the olives came from on the label. Ideally, you want them to come only from one country.

- **Taste it.** Good olive oil should be fruity, bitter (a characteristic of fresh oil), and peppery, which indicates the presence of antioxidants. It should not be musty, vinegary, rancid, or overly buttery.

MEDiTERRANEAN COOKiNG TECHNIQUES AND SHORTCUTS

Cooking is an important experience in the Mediterranean diet. Preparing your own meals means you'll eat healthier, consume fewer calories, save money, and have more control of the ingredients that go in your food. Once you master a few dishes, you'll be preparing your own meals effortlessly. These techniques and shortcuts are used frequently and are simple to master.

VEGETABLE STEWING

The majority of home-cooked Mediterranean dishes are made on the stovetop. Prior to the 1970s, most homes in the Mediterranean did not have ovens, or if they did, they would be outside wood-burning ovens that took time to set up, so stewing on the stovetop was a common way to cook. The first basic step in stewing is to heat olive oil in a pan and then sauté some onions to a point where the onions do not brown but become translucent. The remaining ingredients are then added to the pan, followed by hot water, which should be added only in small amounts. The secret to a good stewed vegetable dish is to create a thick sauce that is not watery, and this is achieved by adding small amounts of water while maintaining a low simmer. The stew should not be boiling; it should just barely bubble.

LATHERA

The Greek word *lathera* means "those cooked in oil." Lathera is a special category of dishes found in Greece, and most stewed vegetable, bean, and rice dishes belong in this category. A generous amount of olive oil is used at the beginning of the dish to add flavor and palatability that might not have been present otherwise. The vegetables are then simmered with tomatoes and herbs until the dish is left, as they say, "with its oil." There should be no water in the dish, just sauce and olive oil.

PAN-ROASTING

Pan-roasting is typically reserved for special occasions and weekends. Meats such as chicken or lamb are often roasted in the oven with olive oil and potatoes or pasta. Beans and vegetables are also often roasted. Beans may be boiled first and then roasted in the oven with herbs and olive oil. When pan-roasting, it's important to be careful with the amount of water you use to avoid a watery or undercooked dish. And water is always added in the corner of a pan and not on top of ingredients in order to avoid washing off the olive oil and seasonings.

BRAISING

Meat in the Mediterranean diet is usually prepared by braising. When braising chicken, beef, or pork, the meat is first browned in olive oil and then cooked in a sauce with vegetables that are added to the pan.

MAKING SAVORY PIES

There's an abundance of savory pies in Greek cuisine. They consist of a crust made with phyllo, which are very thin, unleavened sheets of dough. Several sheets of phyllo are layered to form a crust, filling is then placed on top of the phyllo sheets, and more phyllo sheets are layered on top to cover the filling.

Working with phyllo is easy and forgiving once you know how to do it, but keep the following important points in mind. First, always defrost the phyllo completely in the refrigerator before opening the package. Also, phyllo can dry out fairly quickly, so keep it covered completely with a damp towel when working with it. Finally, most of the surface of the phyllo should be brushed with a thin layer of olive oil to create a crispy and flavorful texture in the crust.

TiME-SAVING SHORTCUTS

One of the concerns I most often hear from people who are just starting the Mediterranean diet is that they think it will require too much time in the kitchen. This is simply not true. Most recipes are easy and relatively quick to make, but some shortcuts will help you save some time in the kitchen without compromising the health benefits or flavor of the recipes.

USE FROZEN VEGETABLES

I'm a big fan of using frozen vegetables. They have a similar nutrient composition to fresh vegetables and are just as healthy. When cooking with frozen vegetables, however, you should make sure any frozen vegetables you buy contain only the vegetables and no other ingredients. You don't have to defrost frozen vegetables when using them in recipes. For a recipe like a vegetable stew, you can just add them after sautéing the onions. I also like to freeze herbs and chopped onions; both are huge time-savers and can help cut prep times dramatically.

USE CANNED BEANS AND TOMATOES

I've found that cooking from dry beans offers a better texture and flavor in many cases, but using canned beans is fine if you wish to do so. You'll avoid the soaking and boiling times associated with cooking dry beans, and you'll only need to add them at the end of the cooking process. Canned, crushed, or chopped tomatoes are also good pantry items to keep on hand and can be used in most of the cooked dishes in this book.

STICK TO A BASIC MENU DURING THE WEEK

When starting a new eating plan, I suggest having a weekday routine with dishes that you have mastered and then using the weekend to experiment with new recipes. This will help ensure that you spend less time in the kitchen during the week, which is when you're likely busier and have less time to cook.

INCORPORATE LEFTOVERS INTO YOUR MEALS

Most Mediterranean dishes actually taste better the next day, particularly vegetable dishes. It is common in Mediterranean culture to consume a vegetable dish for several days. Leftover beans can be added to cold salads, roasted or stewed vegetables can top a slice of whole-grain bread for a hearty bruschetta, or beans can be enjoyed as a side dish the next day.

CREATE A MEZE

In Mediterranean culture we have something called a *meze*, which is an appetizer plate. Homemade meze plates are often made with leftovers and served along with cheese, vegetables, and a few olives. The result? A balanced and delicious meal for which no cooking is required.

Time-Saving Kitchen Tools

Here are some handy kitchen gadgets that can save you time while you cook:

- A salad spinner is great for quickly drying salad ingredients.
- An electric kettle is useful for having hot water always available when you're cooking casseroles and need to add additional hot water to the dish.
- A sharp peeler can quickly remove skin from potatoes, carrots, and cucumbers.
- A microplane grater is perfect for grating cheese or zesting citrus in a pinch.
- An olive oil mister is useful for quickly applying olive oil to recipes.
- A pair of sharp herb scissors can make chopping herbs and greens easier.

CREATING MEALS AND MENUS

Studies have shown that meal planning is associated with healthier eating and lower body weight. It also saves time and money. Follow these tips to plan your weekly meals and make things easier as you embark on this new way of eating.

BALANCING NUTRITION

Any meal plan will balance nutrition over a period of days and not necessarily within every meal, and this is true for the Mediterranean diet. Every meal may not include foods from every food group, but the overall nutrition will be balanced throughout the day and across the week.

BREAKFAST

A breakfast that includes both protein and fiber will keep you feeling full for longer. A typical Mediterranean breakfast includes fruit and a protein, such as yogurt or eggs. A more savory breakfast might include vegetables in place of the fruit.

LUNCH AND DINNER

Lunch and dinner meals should include vegetables or beans, olive oil, and some sort of protein such as cheese, fish, or a nut butter, supplemented with a small amount of carbohydrates, such as bread, or rice, which is typically cooked with the vegetables. Bread is the main starch in the diet, so it's important to choose a whole-grain bread that does not contain any additives, sugars, or unhealthy fats. When eating fish, chicken, or meat, always supplement your meal with extra vegetables.

SNACKS

Snacks on the diet are usually a seasonal fruit. You should avoid only eating snacks that are made mainly from starches, such as crackers or breadsticks, and you should always supplement starches with proteins such as nuts, yogurt, or cheese to help maintain healthy blood sugar levels and keep you feeling full.

CREATING A WEEKLY MENU

Following a few simple steps will help you create your own meal plan.

Make a template to plan your week. Review "The Principles of an Authentic Mediterranean Diet" (pages 16–17), and make a template based on your weekly nutrition requirements. The lower caloric range for a typical meal plan is around 1,700 calories per day, while the higher end is around 2,200 calories per day. A typical weekly meal plan on the Mediterranean diet includes 2 fish meals, at least 2 bean meals, 2 to 3 meals that include pasta or rice along with vegetables or beans, 1 chicken meal, and 1 red meat meal. You can fill in the remaining meals with salads and vegetable dishes, such as casseroles, while supplementing them with a bit of bread and cheese. Once you've settled on the meals to include in your plan, double-check the list to ensure you've included the recommended servings of vegetables, dairy, fruit, and fat.

Choose the recipes. Once you've created an outline for your meal plan, choose the recipes you would like to cook for the week. In addition to factoring in your nutrition needs, you should try to select recipes that fit into your schedule and are based on your tastes. Also, try to include recipes with in-season ingredients. Picking recipes that include common ingredients will save you both money and time, and combining easy, familiar recipes with newer, untested ones helps ensure you're always including recipes and ingredients you enjoy.

Incorporate leftovers into your plan. Most vegetable casseroles will last for 2–3 days, which means you can enjoy them as a main meal on one day and add them as a side on the next. (Savory pies not only make great dinners, but they also make great breakfasts.)

Create a plan that includes new recipes as well as recipes you've tried. It's important to keep things simple when starting a new way of eating. You don't have to cook a different dish every day—start by mastering a few core recipes and include them in your weekly menu plan, and expand your list of recipes as you continue to follow the diet. Include recipes that can be made ahead of time, such as casseroles, savory pies, and roasted dishes.

GENERAL RULES To KEEP IN MIND

Keep these general rules in mind as you put together your weekly eating plan:

- Each serving in the meal plan corresponds to the single serving size indicated in the recipe.
- All fruit are medium-sized, unless specified otherwise.
- If you want to add a 5 fluid ounce (150ml) serving of red wine to a meal, it counts for 120 calories.
- For each serving of alcohol, you should eliminate a half serving from the grain and bread group and a half serving of fat to balance out your caloric levels (see "What to Eat and How Often to Eat It," pages 22–23).
- You can substitute a snack recipe for a main meal if it fits within your menu plan.
- The largest meal of the day should be lunch, but if your schedule does not permit it, you can still make dinner the largest meal of the day.
- Drink at least 50 fluid ounces (1.5l) of water per day.
- Try to drink at least 8 fluid ounces (240ml) of an herbal tea, such as chamomile, thyme, or mountain tea, each day.

Using the Recipes in This Book

The recipes in this book include a wide variety of traditional Mediterranean recipes, as well as some newer Mediterranean-inspired recipes. Several are family favorites that have been passed down from generation to generation, while others are tried-and-true, Mediterranean-inspired recipes that I've developed over the years. Here are a few things to be aware of as you use the recipes:

- Salt is added to the recipes in moderation.
- The majority of recipes are arranged by primary ingredient; however, almost all recipes (with the exception of some meat recipes) include a good amount of vegetables.
- Recipes that are categorized as snacks or breakfast can also be consumed for a main meal. Omelets, for example, are traditionally consumed as a light dinner along with a salad, so don't feel limited by the categories.
- The recommended serving size and the nutrition information at the end of each recipe corresponds to the serving size listed in the recipe.
- The serving sizes for almost all the vegetable dishes are stated as main course serving sizes.
- Each recipe includes a preparation time and cooking time so you can plan your time accordingly.
- Many of the bean recipes require overnight soaking if you are using dry beans.
- When using tomatoes in the cooked dishes, you can use canned or fresh.

TWO-WEEK GETTING STARTED MEDITERRANEAN DIET MEAL PLAN

This 14-day meal plan has been designed to help you get started with the traditional Mediterranean style of eating. It does not need to be followed rigidly, but it is intended to help you learn how to structure your meals throughout the day and incorporate Mediterranean recipes into your weekly eating plan.

WEEK 1

	DAY 1	DAY 2	DAY 3
TOTAL	1,772 calories	1,754 calories	1,745 calories
BREAKFAST	Mediterranean Omelet (p. 40) ½ whole-grain pita	2 Savory Zucchini Muffins (p. 45)	Shakshuka (Poached Egg on Tomatoes with Spices and Onion) (p. 47) 1 slice whole-wheat bread
SNACK	10 medium or 15 small grapes	3 apricots	1 cup plain 2% Greek yogurt topped with 1 chopped peach
LUNCH	Gigantes (Greek Roasted Butter Beans) (p. 59) 1 ounce (30g) feta 1 slice whole-grain bread	Lightened-Up Eggplant Parmigiana (p. 69) 1 slice whole-grain bread	Neapolitan Pasta and Zucchini (p. 90) 1 sliced tomato and 1 sliced cucumber drizzled with 1½ tablespoons olive oil
SNACK	1 sliced apple sprinkled with a pinch of cinnamon 1 cup herbal tea with 1 teaspoon honey	4 Stuffed Dates with Feta, Parmesan, and Pine Nuts (p. 160) 1 cup herbal tea with 1 teaspoon honey	1 orange 1 cup herbal tea with 1 teaspoon honey
DINNER	Panzanella (Tuscan Tomato and Bread Salad) (p. 133)	Tomato Rice (p. 100) topped with ½ cup plain 2% Greek yogurt Dessert: Karithopita (p. 176)	2 servings Sardine and Herb Bruschetta (p. 152) 2 medium carrots, peeled and cut into sticks

DAY 4	DAY 5	DAY 6	DAY 7
1,768 calories	1,757 calories	1,741 calories	1,791 calories
1 cup plain 2% Greek yogurt sprinkled with 2 tablespoons oatmeal or barley flakes and drizzled with 1 teaspoon tahini and 1 teaspoon honey 2 apricots	Kagianas (Scrambled Eggs with Feta and Tomato) (p. 50) 1 slice whole-wheat bread	1 Savory Feta, Spinach, and Red Pepper Muffin (p. 44)	Ricotta and Fruit Bruschetta (p. 42)
1 cup cubed cantaloupe	1 apple	1 banana	2 mandarins
Citrus Mediterranean Salmon with Lemon Caper Sauce (p. 107) 2 zucchini (boiled or steamed) and 1 medium potato (boiled or steamed) drizzled with 1 teaspoon olive oil and the Lemon Caper sauce 2 slices multi-grain crispbread	Greek Chickpeas and Rice with Tahini and Lemon (p. 86)	Greek Roasted Lemon Chicken with Potatoes (p. 123) 1 sliced tomato and 1 sliced cucumber drizzled with 2 teaspoons olive oil	Spiced Oven-Baked Meatballs with Tomato Sauce (p. 120) served over 1 cup brown rice Cabbage and Carrot Salad (p. 137)
1 pear 1 cup herbal tea with 1 teaspoon honey	3 Roasted Stuffed Figs (p. 168) 1 cup herbal tea with 1 teaspoon honey	1 pear 1 cup herbal tea with 1 teaspoon honey	1 apple 1 cup herbal tea with 1 teaspoon honey
Greek-Style Pea Casserole (p. 58) sprinkled with 1 ounce (30g) crumbled feta	Traditional Greek Salad (p. 130) 1 slice whole-wheat bread	Italian Summer Vegetable Barley Salad (p. 149)	Two servings Spanakopita (Greek Spinach Pie) (p. 98)

TWO-WEEK GETTiNG STARTED MEDiTERRANEAN DIET MEAL PLAN

WEEK 2

	DAY 1	**DAY 2**	**DAY 3**
TOTAL	1,728 calories	1,762 calories	1,774 calories
BREAKFAST	Mediterranean-Inspired White Smoothie (p. 51)	Mediterranean Breakfast Pita Sandwich (p. 48) 1 mandarin	Bulgur Wheat Cereal with Apples and Almonds (p. 41)
SNACK	5 No-Mayo Tuna Salad Cucumber Bites (p. 170)	8 large strawberries	½ cup plain, 2% Greek yogurt with 1 teaspoon honey
LUNCH	Lentil Stew (p. 77) 1 ounce (30g) feta	Fasolakia (Greek Green Beans) (p. 60) 1 ounce (30g) feta 1 slice whole-grain bread	Vegetarian Paella (p. 103)
SNACK	1 orange 8 unsalted almonds 1 cup herbal tea with 1 teaspoon honey	1 apple 1 cup herbal tea with 1 teaspoon honey	1 banana 1 cup herbal tea with 1 teaspoon honey
DINNER	Insalata Caprese (Italian Tomato and Mozzarella Salad) (p. 132) 1 slice whole-grain bread	Spanakorizo (Greek Spinach and Rice) (p. 84) 1 ounce (30g) feta 1 slice whole-grain bread	Spanish Sautéed Lemon and Garlic Chicken (p. 124) Mediterranean No-Mayo Potato Salad (p. 145) 1 cup romaine lettuce dressed with 2 teaspoons olive oil and 1 teaspoon lemon juice 1 slice whole-grain crispbread

DAY 4	DAY 5	DAY 6	DAY 7
1,790 calories	1,807 calories	1,800 calories	1,789 calories
1 slice whole-grain bread 1 large hard-boiled egg 1 medium tomato sliced and drizzled with 1 teaspoon olive oil	Tiropita (Greek Cheese Pie) (p. 52) with 1 sliced and lightly salted tomato	1 slice whole-grain bread topped with 2 teaspoons tahini and 1 teaspoon honey	Greek Yogurt Breakfast Bowl with Almonds, Banana, and Tahini (p. 39)
2 mandarins 1 cup herbal tea with 1 teaspoon honey	½ cup plain, 2% Greek yogurt topped with ½ sliced banana	½ cup plain, 2% Greek yogurt topped with 3 chopped apricots	1 cup cubed cantaloupe
Braised Cauliflower (p. 71) 1 ounce (30g) feta 1 slice whole-grain bread	Psari a la Spetsiota (Oven-Roasted Fish with Tomato and Onion) (p. 109) 2 cups whole-grain pasta, topped with the fish sauce 2 cups arugula and five cherry tomatoes, dressed with 1 tbsp olive oil and 1 tsp balsamic vinegar	Hearty Stewed Beef in Tomato Sauce (p. 117) served over 1 cup whole-grain pasta ½ serving of Sicilian Salad (p. 146)	Prasorizo (Greek Leeks and Rice) (p. 85) sprinkled with 1 ounce (30g) crumbled feta 1 slice whole-grain bread
1 cup plain, 2% Greek yogurt topped with 3 tbsp chopped walnuts and 1 tbsp raisins	1 cup cubed watermelon	1 orange 1 cup herbal tea with 1 tsp honey	1 cup herbal tea with 1 tsp honey
2 cups Classic Tabbouleh (p. 129) ½ whole-grain pita bread	Dakos (Cretan Salad) (p. 138)	Beet and Walnut Salad (p. 135) 1 whole-grain pita	Arugula Spinach Salad with Shaved Parmesan (p. 144) 2 slices whole-grain crispbread Dessert: Crispy Apple Phyllo Tart (p. 175)

CHAPTER TWO
BREAKFASTS

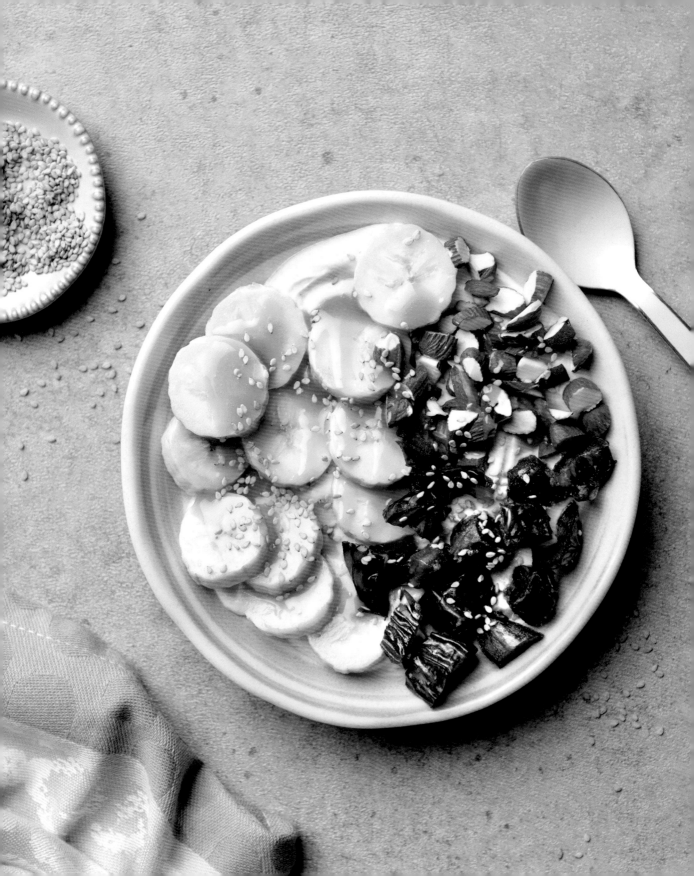

This flavorful yogurt bowl is drizzled with a rich tahini-honey sauce and features banana along with the classic Mediterranean flavors of dates and almonds.

GREEK YOGURT BREAKFAST BOWL
WITH ALMONDS, BANANA, AND TAHINI

 1 SERVING   **5 MINUTES**   **NONE**   **1¼ CUPS**

1 tbsp tahini

1 tsp honey

1½ tsp water

½ cup 2% Greek yogurt

⅛ tsp ground cinnamon

½ medium banana, peeled and sliced

5 unsalted almonds, chopped

2 dried dates, pitted and chopped

⅛ tsp sesame seeds

1 In a small bowl, combine the tahini and honey. Stir, then add the water and continue mixing until the sauce is smooth and velvety. Set aside.

2 In a single-serving bowl, combine the yogurt and cinnamon, then stir.

3 Fan the banana over half the surface of the yogurt, then sprinkle the almonds next to the banana, covering a quarter of the surface. Sprinkle the chopped dates over the remaining quarter of the surface.

4 Drizzle the tahini-honey sauce over the yogurt and fruit, and sprinkle the sesame seeds over the top. Serve promptly. (This recipe is best enjoyed fresh.)

TIP

If you want to reduce the tanginess of the yogurt, combine the tahini-honey sauce with the yogurt prior to topping the bowl with the fruit.

EACH SERVING HAS:

Calories **405**   •   Total fat **14g**   •   Saturated fat **2g**   •   Carbohydrate **62g**   •   Fiber **7g**   •   Protein **9g**

Showcasing the flavors of the Mediterranean, this flavorful and hearty omelet features onion, green pepper, and crumbled feta and is seasoned with fresh mint. It can be enjoyed for breakfast or served with a salad for a light lunch.

MEDITERRANEAN OMELET

 2 SERVINGS   2 MINUTES   11 MINUTES   ½ OMELET

3 eggs

2 tbsp milk

2 tbsp chopped fresh mint

Pinch of salt

Pinch of freshly ground black pepper

1½ tsp extra virgin olive oil

¼ medium onion (any variety), chopped

¼ medium green bell pepper, seeded and chopped

2 tbsp crumbled feta

1 In a medium bowl, whisk the eggs, milk, mint, salt, and black pepper until well combined.

2 Add the olive oil to a medium pan placed over medium heat. When the oil begins to shimmer, add the onions and peppers and sauté for 5 minutes or until the onions are soft.

3 Add the egg mixture to the pan, ensuring it spreads evenly across the bottom of the pan, and sprinkle the feta over the top. Cook for about 3–4 minutes or until the eggs are set on the bottom but still liquidy on top, and then use a rubber spatula to carefully fold the omelet over and in half.

4 Continue cooking for an additional 1–2 minutes or until the eggs are set. To serve, cut in half. Store covered in the refrigerator for up to 3 days.

EACH SERVING HAS:

Calories **177** • Total fat **13g** • Saturated fat **5g** • Carbohydrate **4g** • Fiber **1g** • Protein **11g**

This satisfying and delicious breakfast features juicy, chewy, whole-wheat kernels cooked with apple and raisins, drizzled with honey, and topped with slivered almonds.

BULGUR WHEAT CEREAL
WITH APPLES AND ALMONDS

 1 SERVING   2 MINUTES   23 MINUTES   1 CUP

½ tsp extra virgin olive oil

¼ cup medium-grain uncooked bulgur wheat

½ medium apple (any variety), chopped

1 tbsp raisins

¾ cup hot water

1 tsp honey

1 tbsp slivered or finely chopped almonds

Pinch of ground cinnamon

1 Add the olive oil to a small pan placed over medium heat. When the oil becomes hot, add the bulgur and sauté for 2–3 minutes, stirring frequently with a wooden spoon.

2 Add the apple, raisins, and hot water. When the mixture begins to boil, promptly remove the pan from the heat, cover, and set it aside for 10 minutes. After 10 minutes, add the honey and stir.

3 Top the cereal with the almonds and then sprinkle the cinnamon over the top. Serve warm.

TIP

Bulgur wheat comes in fine, medium, and coarse varieties. The finer variety cooks quicker than the coarser varieties, but a medium variety works best for this recipe.

EACH SERVING HAS:

Calories **295** • Total fat **7g** • Saturated fat **1g** • Carbohydrate **53g** • Fiber **10g** • Protein **6g**

A slightly sweet ricotta spread livens up toast and pairs wonderfully with a pear and banana topping in this delicious morning starter. This high-protein, fiber-rich breakfast will keep you feeling satisfied for hours.

RICOTTA AND FRUIT BRUSCHETTA

 2 SERVINGS   5 MINUTES   NONE   1 SLICE

¼ cup full-fat ricotta cheese

1½ tsp honey, divided

3 drops almond extract

2 slices whole-grain bread, toasted

½ medium banana, peeled and cut into ¼-inch (.5cm) slices

½ medium pear (any variety), thinly sliced

2 tsp chopped walnuts

2 pinches of ground cinnamon

1 In a small bowl, combine the ricotta, ¼ teaspoon honey, and the almond extract. Stir well.

2 Spread 1½ tablespoons of the ricotta mixture over each slice of toast.

3 Divide the pear slices and banana slices equally on top of each slice of toast.

4 Drizzle equal amounts of the remaining honey over each slice, and sprinkle 1 teaspoon of the walnuts over each slice. Top each serving with a pinch of cinnamon.

 TIP
You can make the ricotta mixture ahead of time and store it in the refrigerator for up to 2 days.

EACH SERVING HAS:

Calories **210** • Total fat **7g** • Saturated fat **3g** • Carbohydrate **29g** • Fiber **4g** • Protein **8g**

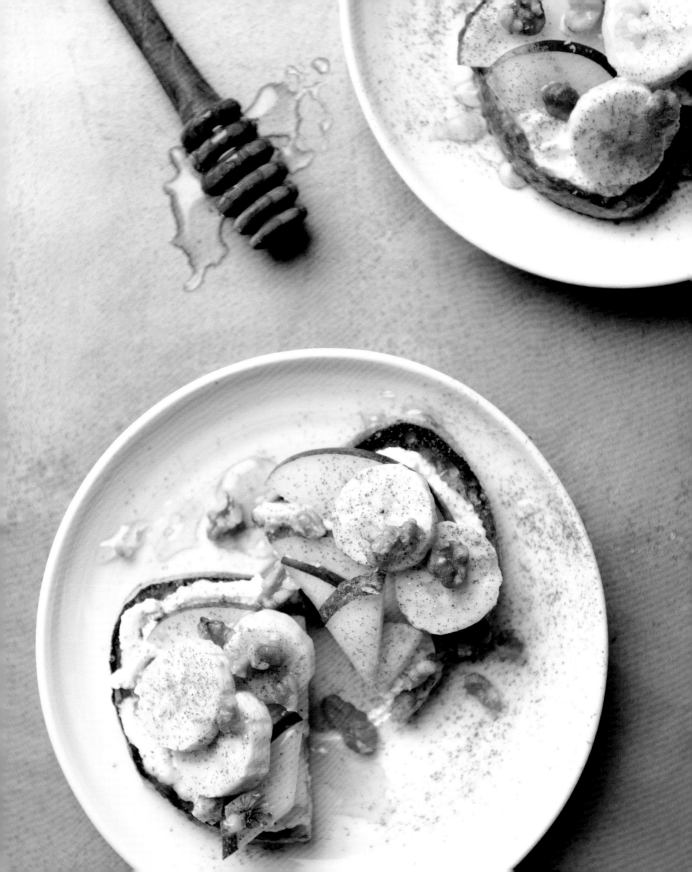

Packed with spinach, sweet red peppers, and feta, these savory muffins are perfect as a snack or for a quick breakfast.

SAVORY FETA, SPINACH, AND RED PEPPER MUFFINS

 12 SERVINGS   10 MINUTES   25 MINUTES   1 MUFFIN

2 cups all-purpose flour

¾ cup whole-wheat flour

¼ cup granulated sugar

2 tsp baking powder

1 tsp paprika

¾ tsp salt

½ cup extra virgin olive oil

2 eggs

¾ cup low-fat 2% milk

¾ cup crumbled feta

1¼ cup fresh baby leaf spinach, thinly sliced

⅓ cup jarred red peppers, drained, patted dry, and chopped

1 Preheat the oven to 375°F (190°C) and line a large muffin pan with 12 muffin liners.

2 In a large bowl, combine the all-purpose flour, whole-wheat flour, sugar, baking powder, paprika, and salt. Mix well.

3 In a medium bowl, whisk the olive oil, eggs, and milk.

4 Add the wet ingredients to the dry ingredients, and use a wooden spoon to stir until the ingredients are just blended and form a thick dough.

5 Add the feta, spinach, and peppers, and mix gently until all the ingredients are incorporated. Evenly divide the mixture among the muffin liners.

6 Transfer to the oven, and bake for 25 minutes or until a toothpick inserted into the middle of a muffin comes out clean.

7 Set the muffins aside to cool for 10 minutes, and remove them from the pan. Store in an airtight container in the refrigerator for up to 3 days. (Remove from the refrigerator 10 minutes before consuming.)

EACH SERVING HAS:

Calories **244** • Total fat **12g** • Saturated fat **3g** • Carbohydrate **27g** • Fiber **2g** • Protein **6g**

These chunky, flourless muffins are seasoned with herbs and contain just the right amount of feta and Parmesan. They're perfect for a savory breakfast treat, an appetizer, or snack anytime of the day.

SAVORY ZUCCHINI MUFFINS

 3 SERVINGS   10 MINUTES   35 MINUTES   2 MUFFINS

1 tbsp extra virgin olive oil plus extra for brushing

2 medium zucchini, grated

⅛ tsp fine sea salt

1 large egg, lightly beaten

1.5oz (40g) crumbled feta

¼ medium onion (any variety), finely chopped

1 tbsp chopped fresh parsley

1 tbsp chopped fresh dill

1 tbsp chopped fresh mint

¼ tsp freshly ground black pepper

3 tbsp unseasoned breadcrumbs

1 tbsp grated Parmesan cheese

1 Preheat the oven to 400°F (200°C), and line a medium muffin pan with 6 muffin liners. Lightly brush the bottoms of the liners with olive oil.

2 Place the grated zucchini in a colander and sprinkle with the sea salt. Set aside for 10 minutes to allow the salt to penetrate.

3 Remove the zucchini from the colander, and place it on a tea towel. Pull the edges of the towel in and then twist and squeeze the towel to remove as much of the water from the zucchini as possible. (This will prevent the muffins from becoming soggy.)

4 In a large bowl, combine the egg, feta, onions, parsley, dill, mint, pepper, and the remaining tablespoon of olive oil. Mix well, and add the zucchini to the bowl. Mix again, and add the breadcrumbs. Use a fork to mash the ingredients until well combined.

5 Divide the mixture among the prepared muffins liners and then sprinkle ½ teaspoon grated Parmesan over each muffin. Transfer to the oven, and bake for 35 minutes or until the muffins turn golden brown.

6 When the baking time is complete, remove the muffins from the oven and set aside to cool for 5 minutes before removing from the pan. Store in an airtight container in the refrigerator for 3 days, or tightly wrap individual muffins in plastic wrap and freeze for up to 3 months.

 TIP

These muffins are best enjoyed warm. To reheat from frozen, unwrap the muffins and place them on a baking sheet in a 350°F (180°C) oven for 10 minutes.

EACH SERVING HAS:

Calories **207** • Total fat **12g** • Saturated fat **5g** • Carbohydrate **13g** • Fiber **3g** • Protein **12g**

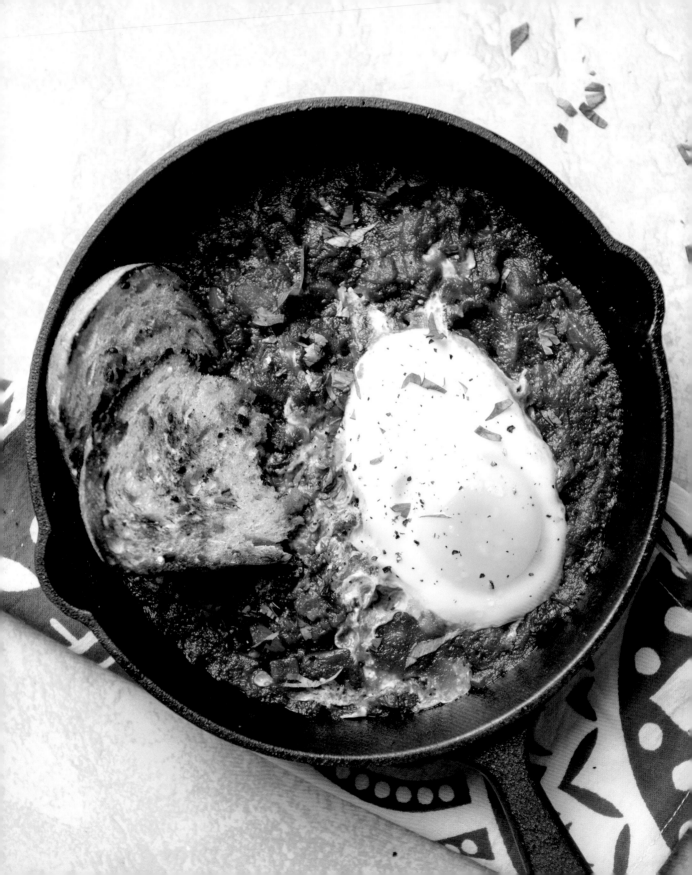

This popular Middle Eastern dish features an egg poached atop a cumin-spiced tomato sauce. It's a traditional recipe that transforms an egg into a flavorful meal.

SHAKSHUKA
(POACHED EGG ON ToMATOeS WiTH SPICES AND ONION)

 1 SERVING   **5 MINUTES**   **13 MINUTES**   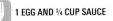 **1 EGG AND ¾ CUP SAUCE**

1 tsp extra virgin olive oil

¼ medium red or white onion, finely chopped

1 cup chopped tomatoes (canned or fresh)

½ tsp ground cumin

½ tsp paprika

1 egg

1 tbsp chopped fresh parsley (for serving)

¼ tsp kosher salt

¼ tsp freshly ground black pepper

1 Place a small pan over medium heat, and add the olive oil. When the oil begins to shimmer, add the onions, and sauté for 3 minutes.

2 In a small bowl, combine the tomatoes, cumin, and paprika. Stir, and pour the tomato mixture into the pan. Stir again and then cover. Bring to a boil, reduce the heat to low, and simmer for 5 minutes.

3 Break the egg on top of the tomato mixture, and continue cooking, uncovered, for 3 minutes. Cover again, and cook for an additional 2 minutes or until the egg is set.

4 Use a spatula to carefully transfer the egg and sauce to a plate. Sprinkle the parsley, kosher salt, and black pepper over the top before serving.

 TIP
Accompany this dish with a slice of whole-grain bread for mopping up the delicious tomato sauce!

EACH SERVING HAS:

Calories **180**   •   Total fat **11g**   •   Saturated fat **3g**   •   Carbohydrate **10g**   •   Fiber **3g**   •   Protein **10g**

Start your day with a pita filled with Mediterranean favorites: eggs, sweet sun-dried tomatoes, tangy feta, crisp cucumbers, and mashed avocado.

MEDITERRANEAN BREAKFAST PITA SANDWICHES

 2 SERVINGS   **5 MINUTES**   **7 MINUTES**   ▮ **½ PITA**

2 eggs

1 small avocado, peeled, halved, and pitted

¼ tsp fresh lemon juice

Pinch of salt

¼ tsp freshly ground black pepper

8-inch (20cm) whole-wheat pocket pita bread, halved

12 ¼-inch (.5cm) thick cucumber slices

6 oil-packed sun-dried tomatoes, rinsed, patted dry, and cut in half

2 tbsp crumbled feta

½ tsp extra virgin olive oil

1 Fill a small saucepan with water and place it over medium heat. When the water is boiling, use a slotted spoon to carefully lower the eggs into the water. Gently boil for 7 minutes, then remove the pan from the heat and transfer the eggs to a bowl of cold water. Set aside.

2 In a small bowl, mash the avocado with a fork and then add the lemon juice and salt. Mash to combine.

3 Peel and slice the eggs, then sprinkle the black pepper over the egg slices.

4 Spread half of the avocado mixture over one side of the pita half. Top the pita half with 1 sliced egg, 6 cucumber slices, and 6 sun-dried tomato pieces.

5 Sprinkle 1 tablespoon crumbled feta over the top and drizzle ¼ teaspoon olive oil over the feta. Repeat with the other pita half. Serve promptly.

EACH SERVING HAS:

Calories **386** • Total fat **20g** • Saturated fat **5g** • Carbohydrate **38g** • Fiber **8g** • Protein **14g**

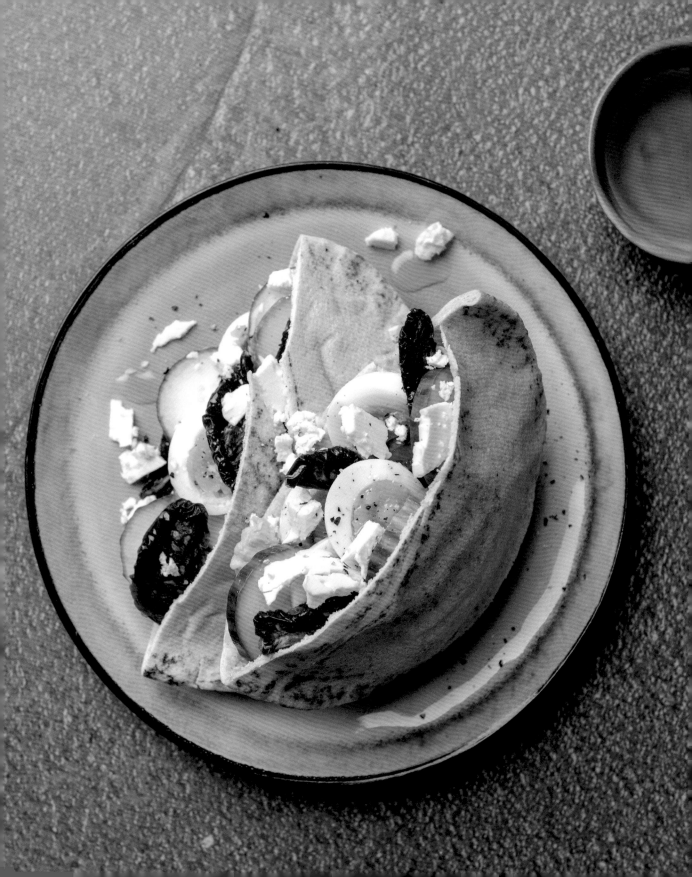

This smooth and creamy dish features scrambled eggs cooked with crushed tomatoes and melted feta. It's a satisfying and flavorful dish that can be eaten for breakfast or lunch.

KAGIANAS
(SCRAMBLED EGGS WITH FETA AND TOMATO)

 1 SERVING   **2 MINUTES**   **13 MINUTES**   **1 CUP**

2 tsp extra virgin olive oil

2 tbsp finely chopped onion (any variety)

¼ tsp fine sea salt, divided

1 medium tomato (any variety), chopped

2 eggs

1oz (30g) crumbled feta

½ tsp dried oregano

1 tsp chopped fresh mint

Pinch of freshly ground black pepper for serving

1 Heat the olive oil in a small pan placed over medium heat. When the oil begins to shimmer, add the onions along with ⅛ teaspoon sea salt. Sauté for about 3 minutes or until the onions are soft.

2 Add the tomatoes, stir, then reduce the heat to low and simmer for 8 minutes or until the mixture thickens.

3 While the tomatoes are cooking, beat the eggs in a small bowl.

4 When the tomatoes have thickened, pour the eggs into the pan and increase the heat to medium. Continue cooking, using a spatula to stir the eggs and tomatoes continuously, for 2–3 minutes or until the eggs are set. Remove the pan from the heat.

5 Add the feta, oregano, and mint, and stir to combine.

6 Transfer to a plate. Top with a pinch of black pepper and the remaining ⅛ teaspoon sea salt. Serve promptly.

 TIP
If desired, you can add other finely chopped vegetables such as leeks, peppers, or greens.

EACH SERVING HAS:

Calories **316** • Total fat **24g** • Saturated fat **8g** • Carbohydrate **8g** • Fiber **2g** • Protein **17g**

Filling and flavorful, with just a touch of sweetness from the honey, this creamy white smoothie will become your go-to recipe for a quick and easy breakfast!

MEDiTERRANEAN-INSPIRED WHiTE SMOOTHIE

 1 SERVING   **5 MINUTES**   **NONE**   🍴 **1⅓ CUPS**

½ medium apple (any variety), peeled, halved, and seeded

5 roasted almonds

½ medium frozen banana, sliced (be sure to peel the banana before freezing)

¼ cup full-fat Greek yogurt

½ cup low-fat 1% milk

¼ tsp ground cinnamon

½ tsp honey

1 Combine all the ingredients in a blender. Process until smooth.

2 Pour into a glass and serve promptly. (This recipe is best consumed fresh.)

EACH SERVING HAS:

Calories **255**   •   Total fat **7g**   •   Saturated fat **2g**   •   Carbohydrate **38**   •   Fiber **5g**   •   Protein **10g**

This savory cheese pie can be enjoyed for breakfast, lunch, or dinner. It features a rich and tangy feta filling wrapped in crispy phyllo dough.

TiROPiTA
(GREEK CHEESE PIE)

 12 SERVINGS   **15 MINUTES**   **45 MINUTES**   **1 PIECE**

1 tbsp extra virgin olive oil plus 3 tbsp for brushing

1lb (450g) crumbled feta

8oz (225g) ricotta cheese

2 tbsp chopped fresh mint, or 1 tbsp dried mint

2 tbsp chopped fresh dill, or 1 tbsp dried dill

¼ tsp freshly ground black pepper

3 eggs

12 (14 x 18-inch/35.5 x 46cm) phyllo sheets, defrosted

1 tsp white sesame seeds

1 Preheat the oven to 350°F (180 C). Brush a 9 × 13-inch (23 × 33cm) casserole dish with olive oil.

2 Combine the feta and ricotta in a large bowl, using a fork to mash the ingredients together. Add the mint, dill, and black pepper, and mix well. In a small bowl, beat the eggs and then add them to the cheese mixture along with 1 tablespoon olive oil. Mix well.

3 Carefully place 1 phyllo sheet in the bottom of the prepared dish. (Keep the rest of the dough covered with a damp towel.) Brush the sheet with olive oil, then place a second phyllo sheet on top of the first and brush with olive oil. Repeat until you have 6 layers of phyllo.

4 Spread the cheese mixture evenly over the phyllo and then fold the excess phyllo edges in and over the mixture.

5 Cover the mixture with 6 more phyllo sheets, repeating the process by placing a single phyllo sheet in the pan and brushing it with olive oil. Roll the excess phyllo in to form an edge around the pie.

6 Brush the top phyllo layer with olive oil and then use a sharp knife to score it into 12 pieces, being careful to cut only through the first 3–4 layers of the phyllo dough. Sprinkle the sesame seeds and a bit of water over the top of the pie.

7 Place the pie on the middle rack of the oven. Bake for 40 minutes or until the phyllo turns a deep golden color. Carefully lift one side of the pie to ensure the bottom crust is baked. If it's baked, move the pan to the bottom rack and bake for an additional 5 minutes.

8 Remove the pie from the oven and set aside to cool for 15 minutes. Use a sharp knife to cut the pie into 12 pieces. Store covered in the refrigerator for up to 3 days.

 TIP

A clear glass casserole dish is ideal for this recipe because you can easily check if the bottom of the crust is done.

EACH SERVING HAS:

Calories **349** • Total fat **24g** • Saturated fat **15g** • Carbohydrate **15g** • Fiber **1g** • Protein **18g**

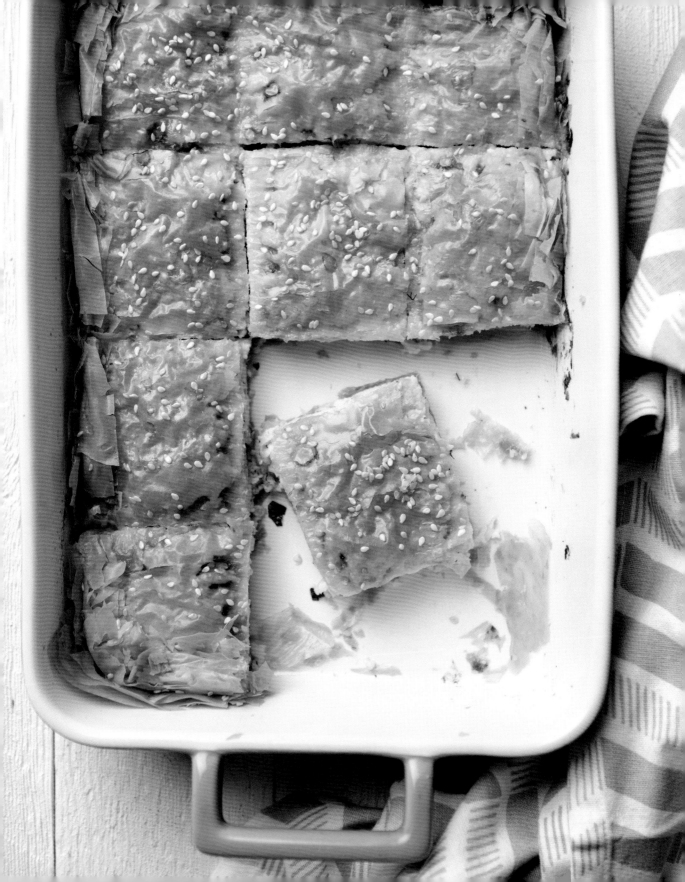

CHAPTER THREE
VEGETABLE AND BEAN ENTRÉES

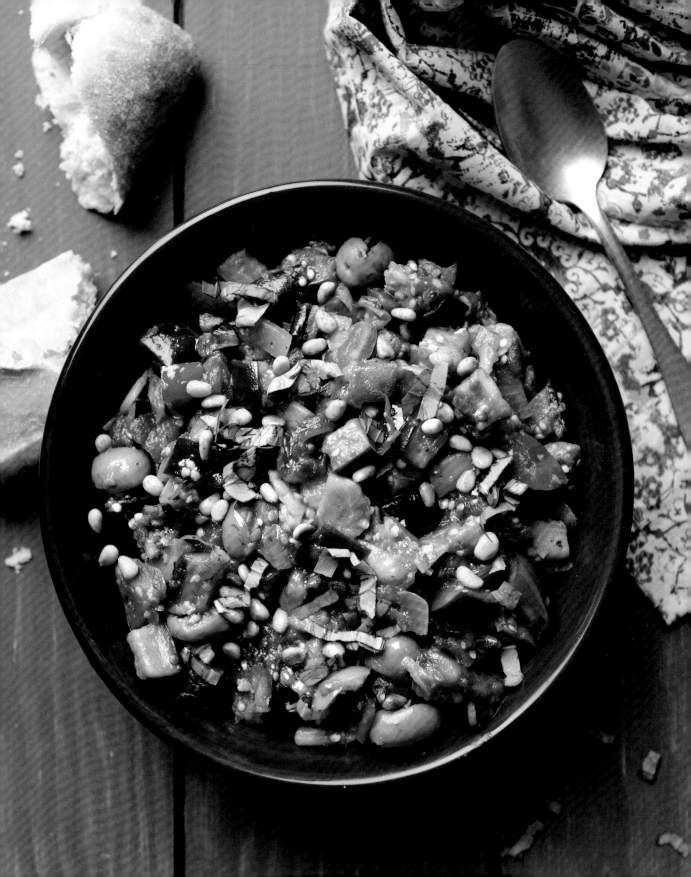

This traditional Sicilian recipe is made of eggplant stewed with tomatoes, onions, capers, and olives. The caramelized eggplant gives this dish a sweet and sour flavor.

CAPONATA
(SICILIAN EGGPLANT)

 4 SERVINGS   **1 HOUR 5 MINUTES**   **40 MINUTES**   **2 CUPS**

3 medium eggplant, cut into ½-inch (1.25cm) cubes (about 1.5lb/680g)

½ tsp fine sea salt

¼ cup extra virgin olive oil

1 medium onion (red or white), chopped

1 tbsp dried oregano

½ cup green olives, pitted and halved

2 tbsp capers, rinsed

3 medium tomatoes (about 15oz/425g), chopped

3 tbsp red wine vinegar

2 tbsp granulated sugar

Salt to taste

Freshly ground black pepper to taste

2 tbsp chopped fresh basil

1 tbsp toasted pine nuts (optional)

1 Place the eggplant in a large colander. Sprinkle ½ teaspoon sea salt over the top and set the eggplant aside to rest for about an hour.

2 Add the olive oil to a large pan over medium heat. When the oil starts to shimmer, add the eggplant and sauté until it starts to turn golden brown, about 5 minutes. Add the onions and continue sautéing until the onions become soft.

3 Add the oregano, olives, capers, and tomatoes (with juices) to the pan. Reduce the heat to medium-low and simmer for about 20–25 minutes.

4 While the onions and tomatoes are cooking, combine the vinegar and sugar in a small bowl. Stir until the sugar is completely dissolved, then add the mixture to the pan. Continue cooking for 2–3 more minutes or until you can no longer smell the vinegar and then remove the pan from the heat.

5 Season the mixture to taste with salt and black pepper. Just prior to serving, top each serving with a sprinkle of chopped basil and toasted pine nuts, if using. Store in the refrigerator for up to 3 days.

 TIP

Soaking the eggplant in salt helps remove the bitterness and also limits the absorption of oil. (This dish is even more delicious served the next day with bread!)

EACH SERVING HAS:

Calories **235** • Total fat **16g** • Saturated fat **2g** • Carbohydrate **20g** • Fiber **7g** • Protein **3g**

Peas are stewed in a rich tomato sauce with carrot and potato in this delicious casserole that can be enjoyed as a main course with some good feta and bread.

GREEK-STYLE PEA CASSEROLE

 3 SERVINGS   **5 MINUTES**   **45 MINUTES**   **1½ CUPS**

⅓ cup extra virgin olive oil

1 medium onion (any variety), diced

1 medium carrot, peeled and sliced

1 medium white potato, peeled and cut into bite-sized pieces

1lb (450g) peas (fresh or frozen)

3 tbsp chopped fresh dill

2 medium tomatoes, grated, or 12oz (340g) canned crushed tomatoes

½ tsp fine sea salt

¼ tsp freshly ground black pepper

½ cup hot water

Salt to taste

1. Add the olive oil to a medium pot over medium heat. When the oil starts to shimmer, add the onions and sauté for 2 minutes. Add the carrots and potatoes, and sauté for 3 more minutes.

2. Add the peas and dill. Stir until the peas are coated in the olive oil.

3. Add the tomatoes, sea salt, black pepper, and hot water. Mix well. Bring to the mixture to a boil, then cover, reduce the heat to low, and simmer for 40 minutes or until the peas and carrots are soft and the casserole has thickened. (Check the water levels intermittently, adding more hot water if the mixture appears to be getting too dry.)

4. Remove the casserole from the heat, uncover, and set aside for 20 minutes. Add salt to taste before serving. Store covered in the refrigerator for up to 3 days.

EACH SERVING HAS:

Calories **423** • Total fat **24g** • Saturated fat **3g** • Carbohydrate **41g** • Fiber **11g** • Protein **12g**

Tender and luscious roasted beans are simmered in tomato sauce with herbs in this filling and satisfying dish that can be served as a main course or an appetizer.

GIGANTES (GREEK RoASTED BUTTER BEANS)

 4 SERVINGS   **10 MINUTES** (plus 10 hours soaking time)   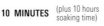 **1 HOUR 45 MINUTES**   **1½ CUPS**

1lb (450g) uncooked gigantes or butter beans

2 bay leaves

¾ cup extra virgin olive oil, divided

2 medium red onions, chopped

4 garlic cloves, thinly sliced

1½ cups canned crushed tomatoes

2 tbsp tomato paste mixed with 2 tbsp water

1 tsp paprika

1 tsp dried oregano

3 tbsp chopped fresh parsley

2 tbsp chopped fresh dill

1 tsp fine sea salt, divided

¼ tsp freshly ground black pepper

Pinch of kosher salt

1 Place the beans in a large bowl and cover with cold water. Soak for 10 hours or overnight, then drain and rinse.

2 When ready to cook, add the beans to a large pot and fill the pot with enough fresh water to cover the beans. Add the bay leaves and place the pot over high heat. Bring the beans to a boil, cover, and reduce the heat to low. Simmer for about 40 minutes to 1 hour or until the beans are soft but not mushy.

3 While the beans are cooking, begin preparing the sauce by adding ¼ cup olive oil to a medium pan placed over medium heat. When the oil begins to shimmer, add the onions and sauté for 5 minutes or until the onions are soft. Add the garlic and sauté for 1 more minute.

4 Add the crushed tomatoes, tomato paste mixture, paprika, oregano, parsley, dill, ½ teaspoon of the sea salt, black pepper, and another ¼ cup of the olive oil, then stir to combine. Let the sauce simmer for about 10 minutes or until it thickens.

5 Preheat the oven to 350° (180°C). When the beans are done cooking, remove them from the heat. Reserve 2 cups of the cooking water, drain the remaining water from the pot, and remove the bay leaves.

6 Add the sauce to the beans, then add the remaining ½ teaspoon of sea salt, and mix gently. Pour the mixture into a baking dish and spread it evenly. Add the reserved cooking water to one corner of the dish and tilt the dish to spread the water across the beans. Drizzle the remaining ¼ cup of olive oil over the beans. Transfer the beans to the oven and bake for 45 minutes or until the sauce is thick and the beans are tender.

7 Remove the beans from the oven and set aside to cool for 15 minutes. Sprinkle a pinch of kosher salt over the top before serving warm or at room temperature. Store covered in the refrigerator for up to 3 days.

EACH SERVING HAS:

Calories **564** • Total fat **42g** • Saturated fat **6g** • Carbohydrate **37g** • Fiber **9g** • Protein **10g**

These tender beans are cooked with potatoes and stewed in tomatoes, parsley, and olive oil. They're so smooth and velvety, they'll melt in your mouth! This dish can be enjoyed as a side but is traditionally consumed as a main course with feta and bread.

FASOLAKIA (GREEK GREEN BEANS)

 2 SERVINGS   **5 MINUTES**    **45 MINUTES**   **2 CUPS**

⅓ cup olive oil (any variety)

1 medium onion (red or white), chopped

1 medium russet or white potato, sliced into ¼-inch (.5cm) thick slices

1lb (450g) green beans (fresh or frozen)

3 medium tomatoes, grated, or 1 (15oz/425g) can crushed tomatoes

¼ cup chopped fresh parsley

1 tsp granulated sugar

½ tsp salt

¼ tsp freshly ground black pepper

1 Add the olive oil a medium pot over medium-low heat. When the oil begins to shimmer, add the onions and sauté until soft, about 5 minutes.

2 Add the potatoes to the pot, and sauté for an additional 2–3 minutes.

3 Add the green beans and stir until the beans are thoroughly coated with the olive oil. Add the tomatoes, parsley, sugar, salt, and black pepper. Stir to combine.

4 Add just enough hot water to the pot to cover half the beans. Cover and simmer for 40 minutes or until there is no water left in the pot and the beans are soft. (Do not allow the beans to boil.)

5 Allow the beans to cool until they're warm or until they reach room temperature, but do not serve hot. Store in refrigerator for up to 3 days.

TIP

If you're serving this recipe as a side instead of a main course, reduce the serving size to 1 cup.

EACH SERVING HAS:

Calories **547** • Total fat **37g** • Saturated fat **5g** • Carbohydrate **44g** • Fiber **12g** • Protein **9g**

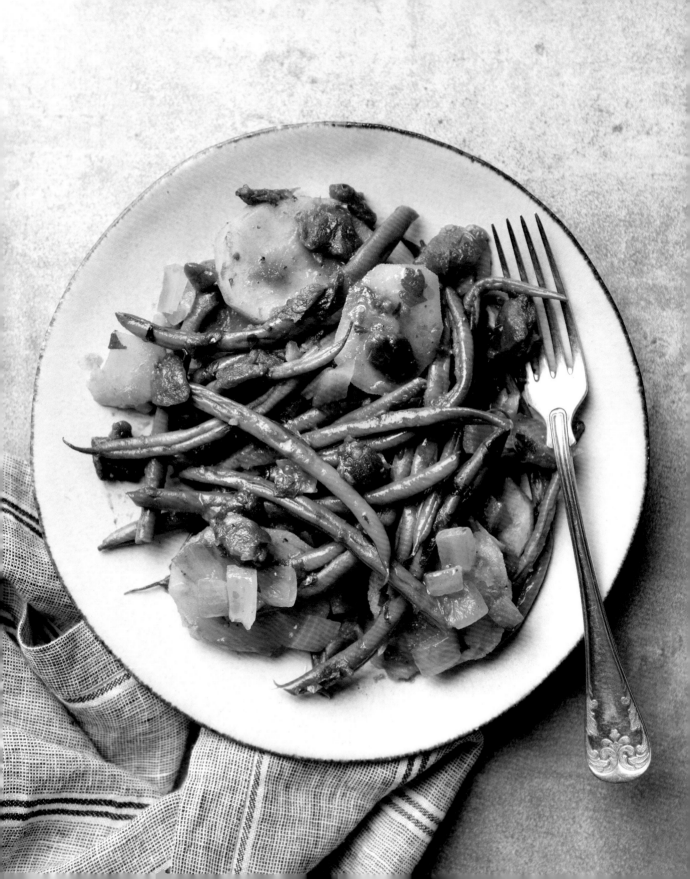

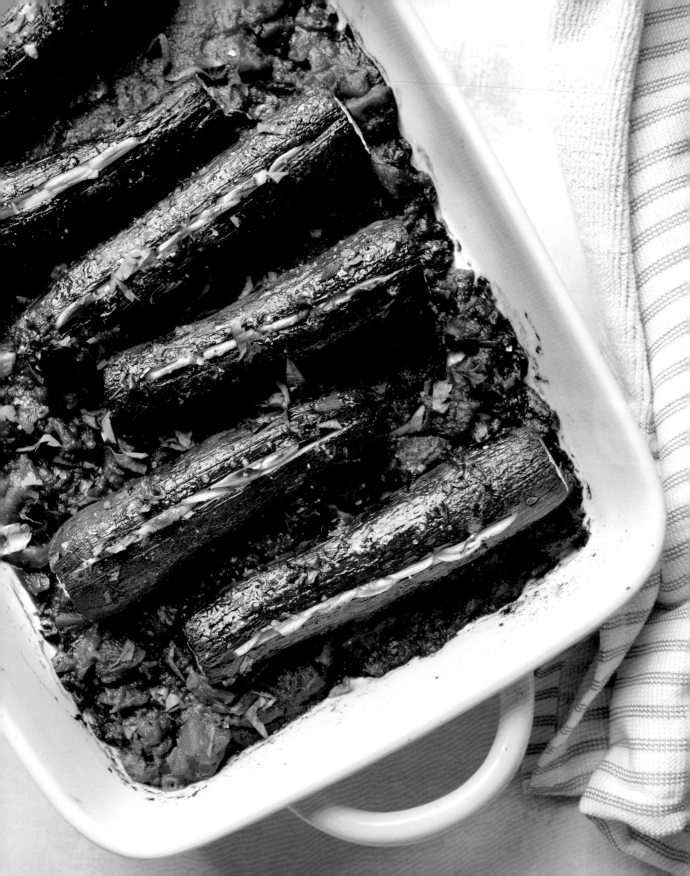

In this traditional Cretan recipe, the zucchini is stuffed with garlic and then oven-roasted with tomatoes, parsley, and olive oil. This delicious recipe is simple to make.

CRETAN ROASTED ZUCCHINI

 6 SERVINGS   **15 MINUTES**   **1 HOUR 15 MINUTES**    **1 ZUCCHINI**

6 small zucchini (no longer than 6 inches [15.25cm]), washed and ends trimmed

3 garlic cloves, thinly sliced

2 medium tomatoes, chopped, or 1 (15oz/425g) can crushed tomatoes

⅓ cup extra virgin olive oil

½ tsp salt

½ tsp freshly ground black pepper

2 tbsp chopped fresh parsley, divided

Coarse sea salt, for serving (optional)

1 Preheat the oven to 350°F (180°C).

2 Make a long, lengthwise slit in each zucchini that reaches about halfway through. (Do not cut the zucchini all the way through.) Stuff each zucchini with the sliced garlic.

3 Transfer the tomatoes to an oven-safe casserole dish, and nestle the zucchini between the tomatoes. Drizzle the olive oil over the zucchini and tomatoes.

4 Sprinkle the salt, black pepper, and 1 tablespoon of the parsley over the zucchini and tomatoes. Turn the zucchini gently so they are covered in the olive oil.

5 Transfer to the oven and cook for 1 hour 15 minutes or until the skins are soft and the edges have browned.

6 Carefully remove the dish from the oven and sprinkle the remaining parsley and sea salt, if using, over the top. Store covered in the refrigerator for up to 3 days.

 TIP
Traditionally, this dish is enjoyed at room temperature and served with bread and feta.

EACH SERVING HAS:

Calories **283** • Total fat **25g** • Saturated fat **4g** • Carbohydrate **10g** • Fiber **6g** • Protein **4g**

A classic Mediterranean staple! Rich and hearty black-eyed peas are cooked in tomatoes along with carrots, onion, and fresh dill, and finished with a squeeze of lemon.

MEDITERRANEAN BLACK-EYED PEA STEW

 2 SERVINGS   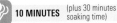 **10 MINUTES** (plus 30 minutes soaking time)    **1 HOUR 10 MINUTES**   **1½ CUPS**

¼ cup extra virgin olive oil

1 large onion (any variety), chopped

2 medium carrots, peeled and thinly sliced

1 cup (about 7oz/ 200g) uncooked black-eyed peas, rinsed and soaked for 30 minutes

1½ cups crushed tomatoes (fresh or canned)

1 bay leaf

2 tbsp finely chopped fresh dill

About 2 cups hot water

½ tsp salt

¼ tsp freshly ground black pepper

1 tbsp finely chopped fresh parsley

1 lemon, for serving

1 Add the olive oil to a medium pot over medium heat. When the oil begins to shimmer, add the onions and carrots and sauté for 5 minutes or until the onions become translucent.

2 Add the black-eyed peas to the pot and sauté for 2 minutes, then add the tomatoes, bay leaf, and dill. Mix well, then add the hot water to the pot. (If needed, add more hot water until the beans are covered in the water by about 1 inch [2.5cm].)

3 Reduce the heat to low and bring the beans to a simmer. Cook for 45 minutes to 1 hour, checking the water levels occasionally and adding more hot water, 2–3 tablespoons at a time, to ensure the beans don't dry out. Remove the beans from the heat when they are soft, and remove the bay leaf. Add the salt and black pepper, and mix well.

4 Transfer to 2 serving bowls and top each serving with ½ tablespoon of the parsley and a squeeze of fresh lemon juice. (You may also accompany this dish with a piece of feta.) Allow to cool completely before storing covered in the refrigerator for up to 2 days.

EACH SERVING HAS:

Calories **448** • Total fat **28g** • Saturated fat **4g** • Carbohydrate **42g** • Fiber **11g** • Protein **7g**

This delicious roasted cauliflower is sweet and nutty, thanks to the caramelization and olive oil. It's topped with Parmesan and freshly ground black pepper.

SHEET PAN CAULIFLOWER
WITH PARMESAN AND GARLIC

 4 SERVINGS   5 MINUTES   40 MINUTES   2 CUPS

1 large head cauliflower (about 6–7 inches/15.25–17.5cm] in diameter), washed and cut into medium florets

2 garlic cloves, minced

⅓ cup extra virgin olive oil

1½ tsp kosher salt

¼ cup grated Parmesan cheese

Freshly ground black pepper to taste

1 Preheat the oven to 400°F (200°C).

2 In a large bowl, combine the cauliflower and garlic. Toss to combine, then add the olive oil and mix well, ensuring the florets are thoroughly coated in the oil.

3 Spread the cauliflower florets in a single layer on a large sheet pan, and drizzle any remaining olive oil over the florets. (Make sure the florets are closely grouped.)

4 Transfer to the oven. Bake for 30–40 minutes or until the florets are golden brown and tender, then carefully remove the pan from the oven.

5 Promptly sprinkle the kosher salt, Parmesan cheese, and black pepper over the top of the florets. Store in the refrigerator for up to 4 days.

 TIP
You can make this dish vegan by removing the cheese. (This is delicious accompanied with some whole-grain bread.)

EACH SERVING HAS:
Calories **251** • Total fat **20g** • Saturated fat **4g** • Carbohydrate **11g** • Fiber **4g** • Protein **6g**

This hearty dish includes white beans, bell peppers, and cherry tomatoes, all roasted in olive oil until moist and tender. Enjoy this dish as is or on bread, bruschetta-style.

ROASTED WHITE BEANS
WITH SUMMER VEGETABLES

3 SERVINGS   **10 MINUTES** (plus 10 hours soaking time)   **1 HOUR 40 MINUTES**   **1¾ CUPS**

1 cup uncooked medium white beans

1 medium red bell pepper, seeded and finely chopped

1 medium green bell pepper, seeded and finely chopped

1 medium onion (any variety), minced in a food processor

1 garlic clove, thinly sliced

½ cup extra virgin olive oil

1 tsp tomato paste diluted with ¼ cup water

1 tbsp dried oregano

1 tsp fine sea salt

¼ tsp freshly ground black pepper

8 cherry tomatoes, halved

¼ cup hot water

1 Place the beans in a medium bowl and cover with water by 2–3 inches (5-7.5cm). Soak overnight or for 10 hours.

2 When ready to cook, drain and rinse the beans, and place them in a large pot. Cover with at least 2 inches (5cm) of water to account for expansion. Place the pot over high heat and bring to a boil, then reduce the heat to medium-low and simmer for about 30 minutes or until the beans are soft but not mushy. Remove from the heat and drain.

3 Preheat the oven to 350°F (180°C). In a large bowl, combine the bell peppers, onions, garlic, cooked beans, olive oil, tomato paste mixture, oregano, sea salt, and black pepper. Toss gently to avoid breaking the beans.

4 Transfer the mixture to a large casserole dish. Place the halved cherry tomatoes on top and then add the hot water to the dish by pouring it into a corner and tilting the dish so that the water spreads across the surface. (Do not pour the water directly over the casserole as this will wash off the olive oil.)

5 Cover the dish with foil and place in the oven to roast for about 1 hour or until the peppers are soft, adding small amounts of hot water, 2 tablespoons at a time, if the beans appear to be drying out. After 1 hour, remove the foil and roast for 10 more minutes.

6 Remove the dish from the oven and set aside to cool for 5 minutes before serving. Store covered in the refrigerator for up to 3 days.

EACH SERVING HAS:

Calories **612**   •   Total fat **37g**   •   Saturated fat **5g**   •   Carbohydrate **52g**   •   Fiber **14g**   •   Protein **18g**

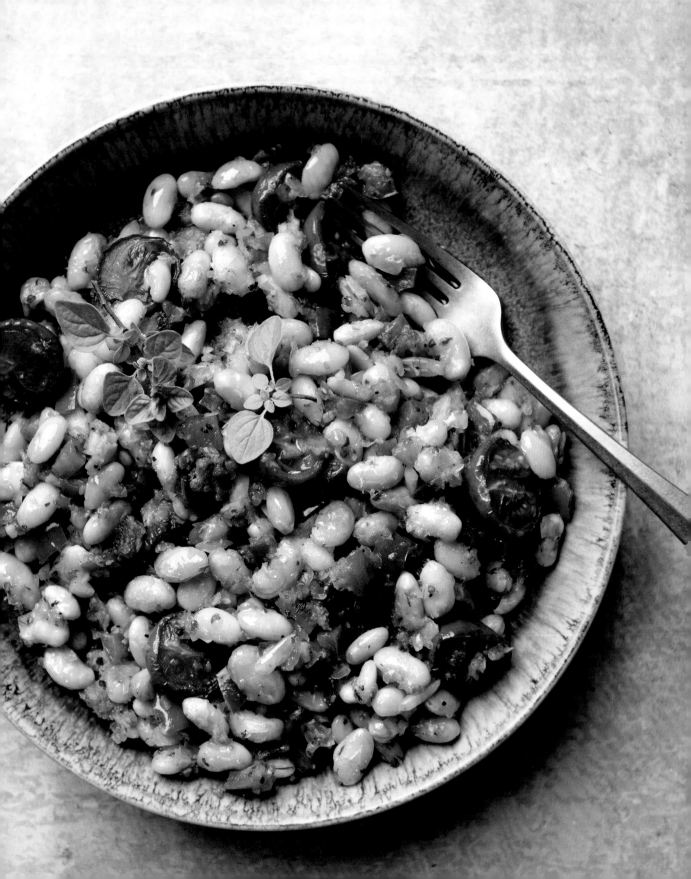

These eggplant are stuffed with caramelized onions and tomatoes, drizzled with olive oil, topped with tangy crumbled feta, and then roasted until tender.

STUFFED EGGPLANT
WITH ONION AND TOMATO

 4 SERVINGS   **10 MINUTES**   **1 HOUR 30 MINUTES**   **1 EGGPLANT**

4 medium, long eggplant, washed and stemmed

6 tbsp extra virgin olive oil, divided, plus 1 tsp for brushing

1⅛ tsp fine sea salt, divided

3 medium red onions, finely chopped

5 garlic cloves, finely chopped

1 tsp granulated sugar

15oz (425g) chopped tomatoes (fresh or canned)

1 cinnamon stick

½ cup chopped fresh parsley

¼ tsp freshly ground black pepper

4 tbsp crumbled feta

4 cherry tomatoes, sliced

1 Preheat the oven to 400°F (200°C). Make 3 end-to-end slits, each about 1 inch (2.5cm) deep, along the length of each eggplant, making sure not to cut completely through. (The slits should be about ¾ inch [2cm] apart.)

2 Place the eggplant in a large baking pan, slit side up. Brush with 1 teaspoon of the olive oil, and season with ⅛ teaspoon of the sea salt. Transfer to the oven and roast for 45 minutes.

3 While the eggplant are roasting, begin preparing the filling by heating 3 tablespoons of the olive oil in a deep pan placed over medium heat. When the oil starts to shimmer, add the onions and garlic and sauté for 3 minutes.

4 Sprinkle the sugar and ¼ teaspoon of the sea salt over the onions. Stir, then reduce the heat to medium-low and cook for 15 minutes or until the onions are caramelized. (Reduce the heat if the onions begin to burn.)

5 Add the tomatoes, cinnamon stick, parsley, black pepper, and remaining ¾ teaspoon of sea salt. Stir, increase the heat to medium, and cook for 3–4 minutes.

6 When the eggplant are done roasting, remove them from the oven, carefully pull the slits open, and stuff each eggplant with the filling.

7 Place the stuffed eggplant snugly in a baking dish. Drizzle the remaining 3 tablespoons of olive oil over the eggplant, ensuring the outsides of the eggplant are coated with the oil. Sprinkle 1 tablespoon of feta over each eggplant and then top with 3–4 slices of cherry tomatoes.

8 Place the stuffed eggplant back in the oven and bake for 15 minutes, then lower the heat to 350°F (180°C) and bake for 30 more minutes. Remove from the oven and set aside to cool for at least 15 minutes before serving. Store covered in the refrigerator for up to 3 days.

EACH SERVING HAS:

Calories **389** • Total fat **24g** • Saturated fat **5g** • Carbohydrate **35g** • Fiber **14g** • Protein **8g**

This lighter take on a traditional Italian dish is rich in flavor and features tender roasted eggplant layered with homemade chunky marinara sauce, mozzarella, and Parmesan.

LIGHTENED-UP EGGPLANT PARMIGIANA

 3 SERVINGS   **10 MINUTES**   **1 HOUR 20 MINUTES**   **2 PIECES**

2 medium globe eggplants, sliced into ¼-inch rounds

2 tbsp extra virgin olive oil, divided

1 tsp fine sea salt, divided

1 medium onion (any variety), diced

1 garlic clove, finely chopped

20oz (565g) canned crushed tomatoes or tomato puree

3 tbsp chopped fresh basil, divided

¼ tsp freshly ground black pepper

7oz (200g) low-moisture mozzarella, thinly sliced or grated

2oz (55g) grated Parmesan cheese

1 Line an oven rack with aluminum foil and preheat the oven to 350°F (180°C).

2 Place the eggplant slices in a large bowl and toss with 1 tablespoon of the olive oil and ½ teaspoon of the sea salt. Arrange the slices on the prepared oven rack. Place the oven rack in the middle position and roast the eggplant for 15–20 minutes or until soft.

3 While the eggplant slices are roasting, heat the remaining tablespoon of olive oil in a medium pan over medium heat. When the oil begins to shimmer, add the onions and sauté for 5 minutes, then add the garlic and sauté for 1 more minute. Add the crushed tomatoes, 1½ tablespoons of the basil, the remaining ½ teaspoon of sea salt, and black pepper. Reduce the heat to low and simmer for 15 minutes, then remove from the heat.

4 When the eggplant slices are done roasting, remove them from the oven. Begin assembling the dish by spreading ½ cup of the tomato sauce over the bottom of a 11 × 7-inch (30 × 20cm) casserole dish. Place a third of the eggplant rounds in a single layer in the dish, overlapping them slightly, if needed. Layer half of the mozzarella on top of the eggplant, then spread ¾ cup tomato sauce over the cheese slices and then sprinkle 2½ tablespoons of the grated Parmesan cheese over the top. Repeat the process with a second layer of eggplant, sauce, and cheese, then add the remaining eggplant in a single layer on top of the cheese. Top with the remaining sauce and then sprinkle the remaining 1½ tablespoons of basil over the top.

5 Bake for 40–45 minutes or until browned, then remove from oven and set aside to cool for 10 minutes before cutting into 6 equal-size pieces and serving. Store covered in the refrigerator for up to 3 days.

EACH SERVING HAS:

Calories **516** • Total fat **31g** • Saturated fat **12g** • Carbohydrate **41g** • Fiber **17g** • Protein **31g**

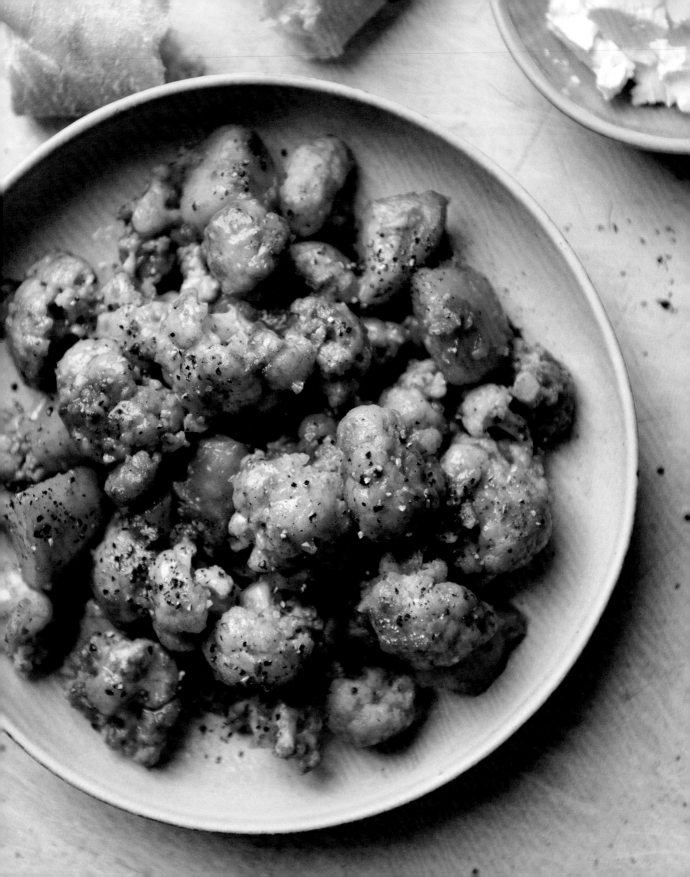

This delicious cauliflower is stewed in olive oil and tomato sauce until tender and flavored with cinnamon, allspice, and clove. Enjoy it as a main course or as an accompaniment to meat or fish.

BRAISED CAULIFLOWER

 3 SERVINGS   **10 MINUTES**   ⏱ **35 MINUTES**   🍴 **1½ CUPS**

½ cup extra virgin olive oil

1 medium head cauliflower (about 2lb/905g), washed and cut into medium-sized florets

1 medium russet or white potato, cut into 1-inch pieces

¼ tsp freshly ground black pepper

3 allspice berries

1 cinnamon stick

3 cloves

2 tbsp tomato paste

1 tsp fine sea salt

¾ cup hot water

1 Add the olive oil to a large pot over medium heat. When the oil begins to shimmer, add the cauliflower, potatoes, black pepper, allspice berries, cinnamon stick, and cloves. Sauté for 4 minutes or until the cauliflower begins to brown.

2 Add the tomato paste and sea salt. Continue heating, using a wooden spoon to swirl the tomato paste around the pan until the color changes to a brick red.

3 Add the hot water and stir gently. Reduce the heat to low, cover, and simmer for about 30 minutes or until the cauliflower is tender and the sauce has thickened. (If the sauce is still watery, remove the lid and simmer until the sauce has thickened.) Remove the allspice berries, cinnamon stick, and cloves.

4 Remove the cauliflower from the heat and set it aside to cool for at least 10 minutes before serving. When ready to serve, transfer the cauliflower to a large serving bowl and spoon the sauce over the top. Store covered in the refrigerator for up to 3 days.

 TIP
This is best enjoyed with feta and a slice of bread for dipping.

EACH SERVING HAS:

Calories **446** • Total fat **37g** • Saturated fat **5g** • Carbohydrate **21g** • Fiber **7g** • Protein **7g**

Beans are cooked with finely chopped carrots, celery, and onion until soft and creamy, then paired with ribbons of egg noodles in this rich and hearty Italian comfort food dish.

VENETIAN-STYLE PASTA E FAGIOLI

2 SERVINGS   **15 MINUTES** (plus 12 hours soaking time)   **50 MINUTES**   **1½ CUPS**

1 cup uncooked borlotti (cranberry) beans or pinto beans

3 tbsp extra virgin olive oil, divided

1 small carrot, finely chopped

½ medium onion (white or red), finely chopped

1 celery stalk, finely chopped

1 bay leaf

1 tbsp tomato paste

2 cups cold water

1 rosemary sprig plus ½ tsp chopped fresh rosemary needles

¼ tsp fine sea salt

¼ tsp freshly ground black pepper plus more to taste

1.5oz (40g) uncooked egg fettuccine or other egg noodles

1 garlic clove, peeled and finely sliced

¼ tsp red pepper flakes

2 tsp grated Parmesan cheese

Pinch of coarse sea salt, for serving

1 Place the beans in a large bowl and cover with cold water by 3 inches (7.5cm) to allow for expansion. Soak for 12 hours or overnight, then drain and rinse.

2 Add 2 tablespoons of the olive oil to a medium pot over medium heat. When the oil begins to shimmer, add the carrot, onions, celery, and bay leaf. Sauté for 3 minutes, then add the tomato paste and continue sautéing and stirring for 2 more minutes.

3 Add the beans, cold water, and rosemary sprig. Cover, bring to a boil, then reduce the heat to low and simmer for 30–40 minutes or until the beans are soft, but not falling apart. Remove the rosemary sprig and bay leaf. Use a slotted spoon to remove about 1 cup of the beans. Set aside.

4 Using an immersion blender, blend the remaining beans in the pot, then add the whole beans back to the pot along with the sea salt and ¼ teaspoon of the black pepper. Increase the heat to medium. When the mixture begins to bubble, add the pasta and cook until done, about 3 minutes.

5 While the pasta is cooking, heat 1 teaspoon of the olive oil in a small pan over medium heat. Add the garlic, red pepper flakes, and chopped rosemary needles. Sauté for 2 minutes, then transfer the mixture to the beans and stir.

6 When the pasta is done cooking, remove from the heat and set aside to cool for 5 minutes before dividing between 2 plates. Drizzle 1 teaspoon of the olive oil and sprinkle 1 teaspoon of the grated Parmesan over each serving. Season with freshly ground pepper to taste and a pinch of coarse sea salt. This dish is best served promptly, but can be stored in the refrigerator for up to 2 days.

TIP
The Venetian version of pasta e fagioli has a thick consistency and is not like a soup.

EACH SERVING HAS:

Calories **660** • Total fat **23g** • Saturated fat **4g** • Carbohydrate **86g** • Fiber **18g** • Protein **27g**

These herbed chickpea patties are chock-full of flavor, plant protein, and fiber. They're baked until golden and finished with a rich tomato sauce.

CHICKPEA PATTiES WiTH TOMATO SAUCE

 2 SERVINGS   **25 MINUTES**   **40 MINUTES**   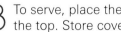 **7 PATTIES**

1½ cups canned chickpeas (about 1 (15oz/425g) can), drained

½ medium onion (any variety), roughly chopped

3 tbsp extra virgin olive oil, divided

1 tbsp chopped fresh basil

2 tbsp chopped fresh mint

1 tbsp chopped fresh cilantro

¼ tsp salt

¼ tsp freshly ground black pepper

¼ tsp ground cumin

1 egg, beaten

2 tbsp unseasoned breadcrumbs

For the tomato sauce

5oz (150g) canned crushed tomatoes

1 tbsp tomato paste

1 garlic clove, minced

1 tbsp extra virgin olive oil

¼ tsp chili powder

¼ tsp paprika

1 cinnamon stick

¼ tsp fine sea salt

Pinch of black pepper

1 Add the chickpeas to a shallow bowl and use a fork to mash until a grainy texture is formed. (It should not be a paste.) Set aside.

2 In a food processor, combine the onion, 1 tablespoon of the olive oil, basil, mint, cilantro, salt, black pepper, and cumin. Pulse until a pulp-like texture is formed.

3 Add the onion-herb mix and beaten egg to the chickpeas and mix with a wooden spoon until well combined. Add the breadcrumbs and mix again, ensuring all the ingredients are well incorporated, until a dough is formed. (The dough should be soft but should hold together enough to form in a ball.) Transfer the dough to the refrigerator to set for 15 minutes.

4 While the dough is setting, make the sauce by combining all the ingredients in a small saucepan over medium heat. Bring the ingredients to a boil and then cover the pan, reduce the heat to low, and simmer for 15 minutes or until the sauce thickens, then remove from the heat, remove the cinnamon stick, and set aside.

5 Preheat the oven to 400°F (200°C) and brush a medium baking pan with 2 teaspoons of the olive oil.

6 Form the patties by shaping 1 tablespoon of the dough into a ball. Place it in the pan and then flatten it. Repeat with the remaining dough to make a total of 14 patties.

7 Brush each patty with 2 teaspoons of olive oil. Bake for 20 minutes, then flip the patties and brush the opposite sides with the remaining 2 teaspoons of olive oil. Bake for 5 more minutes or until golden, then remove from the oven and set aside to cool for 5 minutes.

8 To serve, place the patties on a plate and spoon the tomato sauce over the top. Store covered in the refrigerator for up to 2 days.

EACH SERVING HAS:

Calories **574** • Total fat **31g** • Saturated fat **5g** • Carbohydrate **58g** • Fiber **11g** • Protein **15g**

Crispy potatoes, zucchini, eggplant, onion, tomato, and bell peppers are all roasted together in olive oil. These are perfect with a chunk of feta cheese and fresh bread.

BRIAMI
(SHEET PAN ROASTED VEGETABLES)

 3 SERVINGS   **10 MINUTES**   **2 HOURS**   **2 CUPS**

2 medium potatoes (Yukon Gold or other all-purpose variety), peeled and sliced ¼-inch thick

½ cup cherry tomatoes

1 medium globe eggplant, quartered lengthwise and then cut into ½-inch slices

2 medium zucchini, sliced ¼-inch thick

1 medium red onion, quartered

1 medium green bell pepper, chopped into 1-inch pieces

2 garlic cloves, thinly sliced

½ cup plus 2 tbsp extra virgin olive oil

1 tbsp tomato paste

2 tbsp water

½ tbsp dried mint

1 tbsp dried oregano

¼ cup chopped fresh parsley

1 tsp fine sea salt

⅓ cup hot water

½ tsp coarse sea salt for serving

1 Preheat the oven to 400°F (200°C).

2 Place all the potatoes, tomatoes, eggplant, zucchini, onion, bell pepper, and garlic in a large bowl, and drizzle the olive oil over the top. Use your hands to mix until all the vegetables are coated with the olive oil.

3 In a small bowl, combine the tomato paste, water, mint, oregano, parsley, and sea salt. Stir, add the mixture to the vegetables, and mix.

4 Transfer the vegetables to a sheet pan large enough to hold all the vegetables snugly in a single layer.

5 Pour about ⅓ cup hot water into one corner of the pan and tilt the pan so that the water spreads through the vegetables. (Do not pour the water directly over the vegetables.)

6 Cover the pan with foil and roast for 20 minutes, then lower the oven temperature to 350°F (180°C) and continue roasting for 40 minutes or until you can easily pierce a potato with a fork. (If the vegetables appear to be drying out, add more hot water in small amounts to one corner of the pan.)

7 When the vegetables appear to be cooked, remove the foil and roast for an additional 45 minutes to 1 hour or until the vegetables turn golden brown and crunchy.

8 Remove the vegetables from the oven and set aside to cool for 15 minutes. Sprinkle ½ teaspoon coarse sea salt over the vegetables before serving. Store covered in the refrigerator for up to 3 days.

EACH SERVING HAS:

Calories **484** • Total fat **37g** • Saturated fat **5g** • Carbohydrate **30g** • Fiber **11g** • Protein **8g**

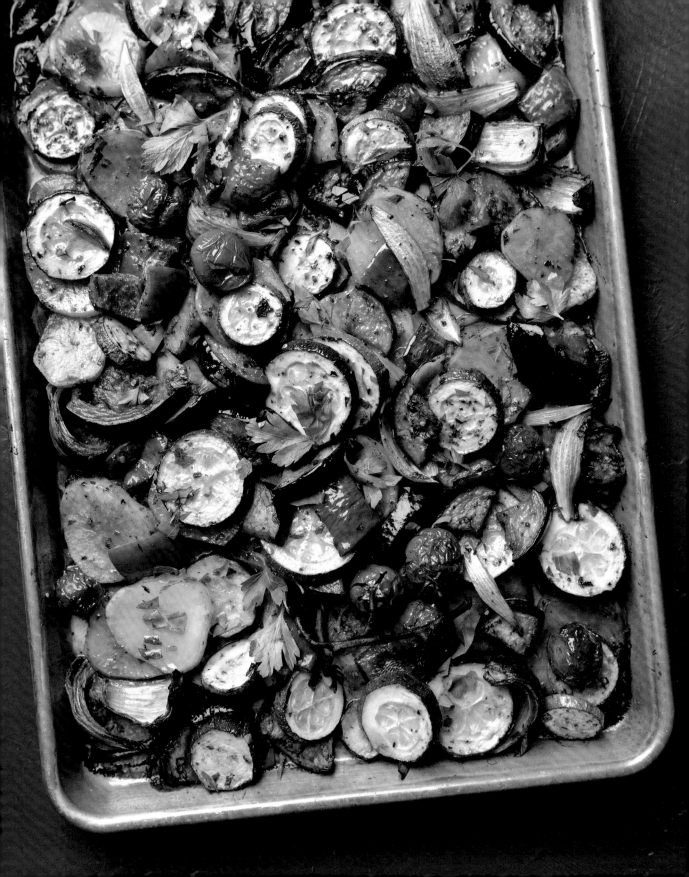

These tender chickpeas are paired with spinach, herbs, and sun-dried tomatoes, and then cooked until all the flavors and textures have melded together.

CHICKPEAS
WITH SPINACH AND SUN-DRIED TOMATOES

 3 SERVINGS   **10 MINUTES** (plus 12 hours soaking time)   **2½ HOURS**   **1⅓ CUPS**

½lb (225g) uncooked chickpeas

4 tbsp extra virgin olive oil, divided

2 spring onions (white parts only), sliced

1 small onion (any variety), diced

1lb (450g) fresh spinach, washed and chopped

½ cup white wine

½ cup sun-dried tomatoes (packed in oil), drained, rinsed, and chopped

1 tbsp chopped fresh mint

1 tbsp chopped fresh dill

6 tbsp fresh lemon juice, divided

¼ tsp freshly ground black pepper

¾ tsp fine sea salt

1 Place the chickpeas in a large bowl and cover with cold water by 3 inches (7.5cm) to allow for expansion. Soak overnight or for 12 hours.

2 When ready to cook, drain and rinse the chickpeas. Place them in a large pot and cover with cold water. Place the pot over high heat and bring to a boil (using a slotted spoon to remove any foam), then reduce the heat to low and simmer until the chickpeas are tender but not falling apart, about 1 to 1½ hours, checking the chickpeas every 30 minutes to ensure they aren't overcooking. Use the slotted spoon to transfer the chickpeas a medium bowl and then reserve the cooking water. Set aside.

3 In a deep pan, heat 3 tablespoons of the olive oil over medium heat. When the oil begins to shimmer, add the spring onions and diced onions, and sauté for 5 minutes or until soft, then add the spinach. Toss and continue cooking for 5–7 minutes or until the spinach has wilted. Add the wine and continue cooking for 2 minutes or until the liquid has evaporated.

4 Add the cooked chickpeas, sun-dried tomatoes, mint, dill, 3 tablespoons of the lemon juice, black pepper, and 1½ cups of the chickpea cooking water. Bring the mixture to a boil and then reduce the heat to low and simmer for 30–45 minutes or until the liquid has been absorbed and the chickpeas have thickened, adding more water as needed if the chickpeas appear to be too dry. About 5 minutes before removing the chickpeas from the heat, add the remaining 1 tablespoon of olive oil, a tablespoon of the lemon juice, and the sea salt. Mix well, then remove the pan from the heat, keeping it covered, and set aside to rest for 5 minutes.

5 Divide the mixture between three bowls and top each serving with 1 tablespoon of the lemon juice. Store covered in the refrigerator for up to 3 days.

EACH SERVING HAS:

Calories **528** • Total fat **24g** • Saturated fat **3g** • Carbohydrate **59g** • Fiber **18g** • Protein **21g**

A Greek favorite! This classic stew is simple yet comforting, and intended to be enjoyed year-round. The lentils are cooked until tender with a hint of garlic and then finished with extra virgin olive oil and red wine vinegar.

LeNTiL STEW

 4 SERVINGS   **10 MINUTES**   **30 MINUTES**   **1½ CUPS**

2 tbsp extra virgin olive oil plus 3 tbsp for serving

2 medium onions (red or white), chopped

2 garlic cloves, halved

1 bay leaf

1lb (450g) uncooked brown lentils, rinsed and drained

1 cup canned crushed tomatoes

4 cups hot water

½ tsp fine sea salt

¼ tsp freshly ground black pepper

1 tsp dried oregano

4 tbsp red wine vinegar

Pinch of coarse sea salt to serve

1 Add 2 tablespoons of the olive oil to a large pot over medium heat. When the oil begins to shimmer, add the onions and sauté for 3 minutes or until soft.

2 Add the garlic, bay leaf, and lentils to the pot. Continue cooking, stirring continuously, for 1 minute, then add the crushed tomatoes and continue cooking for 1 more minute.

3 Add the hot water and bring the mixture to a boil, then cover, reduce the heat to low, and simmer for 25 minutes. (Do not add any salt during the cooking as this can harden the lentils.) Halfway through the cooking time, check the lentils. If the water is running low, add more hot water as needed (½ cup at a time) and continue simmering until the lentils are soft and have thickened, then remove the pot from heat.

4 Add the sea salt and black pepper, mix well, then cover and set aside to cool for 15 minutes.

5 When the lentils have cooled, top each serving with 2 teaspoons of olive oil, a pinch of dried oregano, and 1 tablespoon of red wine vinegar. Divide a pinch of coarse sea salt across all servings. Store in the refrigerator for up to 3 days.

 TIP

This stew is delicious when topped with feta, Kalamata olives, or anchovies.

EACH SERVING HAS:

Calories **294** • Total fat **12g** • Saturated fat **2g** • Carbohydrate **34g** • Fiber **16g** • Protein **13g**

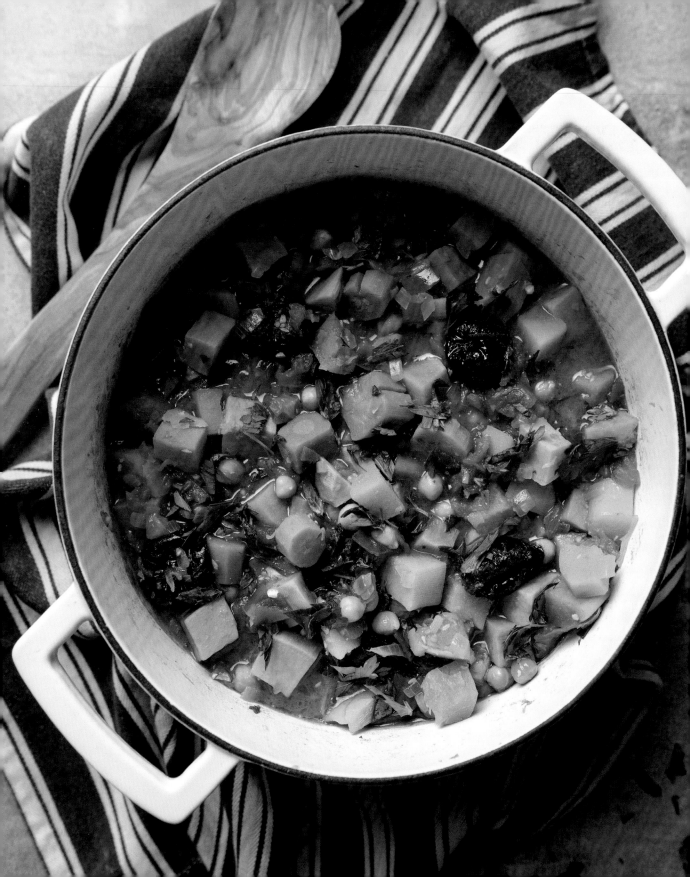

This colorful stew combines sweet and savory flavors. Squash, sweet potato, and prunes, along with spices and chickpeas, give this dish both personality and flavor.

SWEET PoTATo AND CHICKPEA MOROCCAN STEW

  4 SERVINGS    10 MINUTES   40 MINUTES   1½ CUPS

6 tbsp extra virgin olive oil

2 medium red or white onions, finely chopped

6 garlic cloves, minced

3 medium carrots (about 8oz/225g), peeled and cubed

1 tsp ground cumin

1 tsp ground coriander

½ tsp smoked paprika

½ tsp ground turmeric

1 cinnamon stick

½lb (225g) butternut squash, peeled and cut into ½-inch cubes

2 medium sweet potatoes, peeled and cut into ½-inch cubes

4oz (115g) prunes, pitted

4 tomatoes (any variety), chopped, or 20oz (565g) canned chopped tomatoes

14fl oz (415ml) vegetable broth

14oz (400g) canned chickpeas

½ cup chopped fresh parsley, for serving

1 Place a deep pan over medium heat and add the olive oil. When the oil is shimmering, add the onions and sauté for 5 minutes, then add the garlic and carrots, and sauté for 1 more minute.

2 Add the cumin, coriander, paprika, turmeric, and cinnamon stick. Continue cooking, stirring continuously, for 1 minute, then add the squash, sweet potatoes, prunes, tomatoes, and vegetable broth. Stir, cover, then reduce the heat to low and simmer for 20 minutes, stirring occasionally and checking the water levels, until the vegetables are cooked through. (If the stew appears to be drying out, add small amounts of hot water until the stew is thick.)

3 Add the chickpeas to the pan, stir, and continue simmering for 10 more minutes, adding more water if necessary. Remove the pan from the heat, discard the cinnamon stick, and set the stew aside to cool for 10 minutes.

4 When ready to serve, sprinkle the chopped parsley over the top of the stew. Store covered in the refrigerator for up to 4 days.

 TIP

Because this recipe has so many ingredients, it can be helpful to measure out everything before starting the cooking process.

EACH SERVING HAS:

Calories **516** • Total fat **22g** • Saturated fat **3g** • Carbohydrate **70g** • Fiber **13g** • Protein **10g**

CHAPTER FOUR

PASTA, RICE, AND SAVORY PIE ENTRÉES

A classic favorite combination: rice and beans with a Mediterranean twist. The rice is cooked until smooth and paired with lentils, tomatoes, garlic, carrots, and onions.

FAKORIZO
(GREEK LENTILS WITH VEGETABLES AND RICE)

 2 SERVINGS   10 MINUTES 45 MINUTES  1½ CUPS

½ cup uncooked brown lentils, rinsed and drained

3 cups hot water, divided

1 bay leaf

3 tbsp extra virgin olive oil

1 medium onion (any variety), chopped

2 medium carrots, peeled and diced

2 garlic cloves, minced

½ cup uncooked medium-grain rice

1 tsp fine sea salt

¼ tsp freshly ground black pepper

1 medium tomato (any variety), diced

Chopped fresh parsley, for serving

1 Place the lentils in a medium pot along with 1½ cups of the hot water and bay leaf. Bring to a boil over medium-high heat, then reduce the heat to low and simmer for 20 minutes or until the lentils are soft but not mushy. Drain and set aside.

2 Add the olive oil to a large, deep pan placed over medium heat. When the oil begins to shimmer, add the onions and sauté for 5 minutes or until translucent. Add the carrots and sauté 2–3 minutes more, then add the garlic and sauté for an additional 30 seconds.

3 Add the rice and stir until the rice is coated in the olive oil. Add the lentils, sea salt, and black pepper, and mix well.

4 Add the tomato and remaining 1½ cups hot water. Cover, reduce the heat to low, and simmer for about 15 minutes or until the rice is cooked and the water is absorbed, adding more hot water as needed.

5 Remove the pan from heat and fluff the lentils with a fork. Sprinkle the parsley over the top to serve. Store covered in the refrigerator for up to 3 days.

EACH SERVING HAS:

Calories **418** • Total fat **21g** • Saturated fat **3g** • Carbohydrate **53g** • Fiber **4g** • Protein **5g**

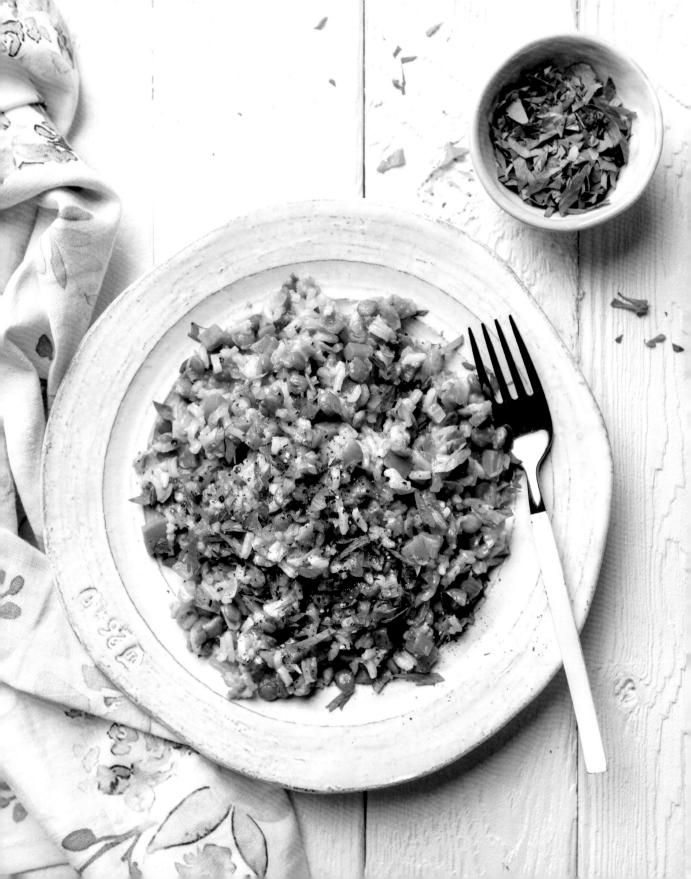

This healthy and delicious comfort food dish features soft and creamy spinach cooked with rice, seasoned with herbs, and finished with a squeeze of lemon.

SPANAKORIZO
(GREEK SPINACH AND RICE)

 2 SERVINGS   5 MINUTES   27 MINUTES   2 CUPS

3½ tbsp extra virgin olive oil, divided

1lb (450g) fresh spinach, rinsed and torn into large pieces

2 tbsp fresh lemon juice plus juice of ½ lemon, for serving

1 medium red onion, chopped

1 tsp dried mint

2 tbsp chopped fresh dill

⅓ cup uncooked medium-grain rice

⅔ cup hot water

½ tsp fine sea salt

¼ tsp freshly ground black pepper

1 Add 1½ teaspoons of olive oil to a deep pan over medium heat. When the oils starts to shimmer, add the spinach and 2 tablespoons lemon juice. Using tongs, toss the spinach until it's wilted and develops a bright green color, about 2–3 minutes, then transfer to a colander and set aside to drain.

2 In a separate large pot placed over medium heat, combine the onions with 2 tablespoons of the olive oil. Sauté until the onions are soft, about 3 minutes.

3 Add the cooked spinach, mint, dill, and rice to the pot and then stir to coat the spinach and rice in the olive oil. Continue sautéing for 1 minute, then add the hot water, sea salt, and black pepper. Stir, then increase the heat slightly and bring the mixture to a boil.

4 Once the mixture comes to a boil, reduce the heat to low and simmer for 20 minutes or until the rice is soft, adding more warm water as needed if the rice becomes too dry.

5 Serve warm or at room temperature with a squeeze of lemon juice and 1½ teaspoons of the olive oil drizzled over each serving. Store covered in the refrigerator for up to 3 days.

TIP

This can be enjoyed as a vegan dish, but it also pairs perfectly with a small piece of feta.

EACH SERVING HAS:

Calories **431** • Total fat **25g** • Saturated fat **4g** • Carbohydrate **42g** • Fiber **7g** • Protein **10g**

This traditional, popular Greek vegan dish is made with leeks and rice. It's rich, sweet, and creamy thanks to the caramelized leeks.

PRASORIZO
(GREEK LEEKS AND RICE)

 2 SERVINGS   **10 MINUTES**   **30 MINUTES**   **1¾ CUPS**

2 cups sliced leeks, white and pale green parts only, cut into ½-inch (1.25cm) slices

⅓ cup extra virgin olive oil

2 tbsp chopped fresh dill

2 tsp tomato paste

½ tsp fine sea salt

¼ tsp freshly ground black pepper plus extra to taste

½ cup uncooked medium-grain rice

1½ cups hot water

Juice of 1 lemon

1 Fill a large pot with water and bring to a boil over high heat. Once the water is boiling, place the leeks in the pot and boil for 2–3 minutes. Drain and set aside.

2 Add the olive oil to a medium pot over medium-low heat. When the oil begins to shimmer, add the leeks and sauté until soft, about 6–7 minutes. (Do not allow the leeks to brown.)

3 Add the dill, tomato paste, sea salt, and black pepper. Stir a few times, then add the rice and mix until the rice is coated with the oil. Add the hot water and mix well.

4 Cover the pot and reduce the heat to low. Simmer for about 20 minutes or until the rice is soft, checking the rice regularly and adding more hot water as needed. When the rice is soft, turn off the heat—keeping the pot covered—and set aside for 10 minutes.

5 Squeeze the lemon over the top, and season with black pepper to taste. Store covered in the refrigerator for up to 3 days.

EACH SERVING HAS:

Calories **496** • Total fat **36g** • Saturated fat **5g** • Carbohydrate **39g** • Fiber **2g** • Protein **4g**

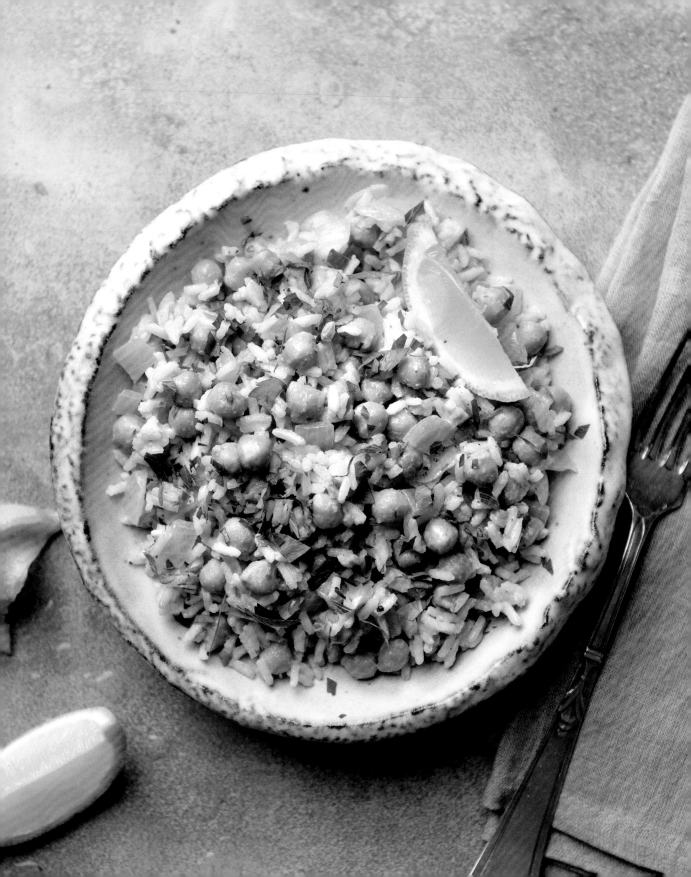

The rice in this comforting and hearty one-pot dish is cooked in lemon and tahini until soft and creamy, and then combined with chickpeas.

GREEK CHICKPEAS AND RICE
WITH TAHINI AND LEMON

 2 SERVINGS   **10 MINUTES** (plus 12 hours soaking time)   **1 HOUR 45 MINUTES**   **2 CUPS**

¾ cup uncooked chickpeas

1 tbsp tahini

3 tbsp fresh lemon juice plus juice of 1 lemon for serving

4 tbsp water

2 tbsp extra virgin olive oil

1 medium onion (any variety), chopped

1 garlic clove, minced

¾ cup uncooked medium-grain rice

¾ tsp fine sea salt

½ tsp freshly ground black pepper

1 bay leaf

2½ cups reserved cooking water

4 tsp chopped fresh parsley

1 Place the chickpeas in a large bowl and cover with cold water by 3 inches to allow for expansion. Soak overnight or for 12 hours.

2 In a small bowl, combine the tahini with the lemon juice and 4 tablespoons of water. Whisk with a fork. Set aside.

3 When ready to cook, drain and rinse the chickpeas. Fill a large pot with cold water, place it over high heat, and add the chickpeas. Bring to a boil (removing any foam with a slotted spoon), then reduce the heat to medium-low and simmer until the chickpeas are tender but not falling apart, about 60–90 minutes. (Some chickpeas will cook faster, so begin checking after 30 minutes.) Reserve 2½ cups of the cooking water and then drain the chickpeas. Set aside.

4 Add the olive oil to a medium pot placed over medium heat. When the oil begins to shimmer, add the onions and sauté for 4–5 minutes or until the onions are soft. Add the garlic and sauté for more 1 minute, then add the rice and stir until the rice is coated in the oil.

5 Add the tahini-lemon juice mixture to the pot, followed by the sea salt, black pepper, bay leaf, and 1½ cups of the cooking water (if using canned chickpeas, use 1½ cups tap water instead). Reduce the heat to medium-low and simmer for about 10 minutes, then add the chickpeas and continue simmering until the rice is cooked and the water has been absorbed, about 10 minutes, then remove the pot from the heat. (Add more hot water in small amounts if the mixture appears to be too dry.) Remove the pot from the heat.

6 Discard the bay leaf and transfer the mixture to two bowls. Squeeze half a lemon over each serving, then sprinkle 2 teaspoons of the parsley over each serving. Store covered in the refrigerator for up to 3 days.

EACH SERVING HAS:
Calories **734** • Total fat **22g** • Saturated fat **3g** • Carbohydrate **111g** • Fiber **10g** • Protein **21g**

This tasty pasta is full of Mediterranean flavor, featuring spinach and tomatoes cooked to perfection along with hints of garlic and feta.

ROTINI WITH SPINACH, CHERRY TOMATOES, AND FETA

 2 SERVINGS   **5 MINUTES**   **30 MINUTES**   **1½ CUPS**

6oz (170g) uncooked rotini pasta (penne pasta will also work)

1 garlic clove, minced

3 tbsp extra virgin olive oil, divided

1½ cups (about 9oz [255g]) cherry tomatoes, halved and divided

9oz (255g) baby leaf spinach, washed and chopped

1.5oz (43g) crumbled feta, divided

Kosher salt, to taste

Freshly ground black pepper, to taste

1 Cook the pasta according to the package instructions, reserving ½ cup of the cooking water. Drain and set aside.

2 While the pasta is cooking, combine the garlic with 2 tablespoons of the olive oil in a small bowl. Set aside.

3 Add the remaining tablespoon of olive oil to a medium pan placed over medium heat and then add 1 cup of the tomatoes. Cook for 2–3 minutes, then use a fork to mash lightly.

4 Add the spinach to the pan and continue cooking, stirring occasionally, until the spinach is wilted and the liquid is absorbed, about 4–5 minutes.

5 Transfer the cooked pasta to the pan with the spinach and tomatoes. Add 3 tablespoons of the pasta water, the garlic and olive oil mixture, and 1 ounce of the crumbled feta. Increase the heat to high and cook for 1 minute.

6 Top with the remaining cherry tomatoes and feta, and season to taste with kosher salt and black pepper. Store covered in the refrigerator for up to 2 days.

TIP

To make this dish vegan, omit the feta. (This dish is wonderful accompanied with a tossed green salad.)

EACH SERVING HAS:

Calories **613**   •   Total fat **27g**   •   Saturated fat **6g**   •   Carbohydrate **74g**   •   Fiber **7g**   •   Protein **19g**

An incredibly easy recipe to make, this flavorful pie features shredded zucchini along with red bell peppers, onions, mint, and feta. It's perfect for breakfast, lunch, or a snack.

CRUSTLESS SAVORY ZUCCHINI AND FETA PIE

 6 SERVINGS   30 MINUTES   1 HOUR   1 SLICE

4 medium zucchini (about 1lb [450g])

¾ tsp fine sea salt, divided

2 eggs

1 cup 2% Greek yogurt

⅓ cup extra virgin olive oil plus 1 tsp for brushing

1 cup self-rising flour

1 medium red bell pepper, chopped

½ medium onion (any variety), chopped

⅓ cup chopped fresh mint

½ tsp freshly ground black pepper

7oz (200g) crumbed feta, divided

4 tsp unseasoned breadcrumbs, divided

1 Use the largest holes of a box grater to grate the zucchini, then transfer to a colander. Sprinkle with ½ teaspoon of the sea salt and set aside for 30 minutes to drain.

2 While the zucchini is draining, whisk the eggs in a large bowl, then add the Greek yogurt and ⅓ cup of the olive oil and mix well. Add the flour and mix again until well combined.

3 When the zucchini is done draining, place it in a tea towel or thin kitchen towel, bring the ends of the towel together, and twist to squeeze out as much of the liquid as possible.

4 Preheat the oven to 350°F (180°C). Combine the grated zucchini, bell pepper, onion, mint, black pepper, remaining ¼ teaspoon of the sea salt, and all but 2 tablespoons of the crumbled feta in a separate large bowl. Mix well. Add the zucchini mixture to the flour mixture and mix well.

5 Brush a 12-inch (30.5cm) round baking pan with 1 teaspoon of the olive oil, making sure to brush the sides of the pan as well. Sprinkle 2 teaspoons of the breadcrumbs into the bottom of the pan.

6 Transfer the zucchini-flour mixture to the pan and use a spatula to spread the mixture into an even layer. Sprinkle the remaining 2 tablespoons of crumbled feta over the top followed by the remaining 2 teaspoons of breadcrumbs.

7 Bake for 1 hour or until the pie is set and the top is golden brown. Set aside to cool for 20 minutes before cutting into 6 slices. Store covered in the refrigerator for up to 2 days.

EACH SERVING HAS:

Calories **211** • Total fat **9g** • Saturated fat **6g** • Carbohydrate **22g** • Fiber **2g** • Protein **11g**

In this traditional Italian pasta dish, zucchini is cooked with pasta and olive oil until it's creamy and velvety, giving it a risotto-like texture. This healthy recipe will become a favorite comfort food.

NEAPOLITAN PASTA AND ZUCCHINI

 3 SERVINGS   5 MINUTES   🕐 28 MINUTES   🍴 2 CUPS

⅓ cup extra virgin olive oil

1 large onion (any variety), diced

1 tsp fine sea salt, divided

2 large zucchini (about 1¾lb [795g]), quartered lengthwise and cut into ½-inch pieces

10oz (285g) uncooked spaghetti, broken into 1-inch pieces

2 tbsp grated Parmesan cheese

2oz (55g) grated or shaved Parmesan cheese for serving

½ tsp freshly ground black pepper

1 Add the olive oil to a medium pot over medium heat. When the oil begins to shimmer, add the onions and ¼ teaspoon of the sea salt. Sauté for 3 minutes, add the zucchini, and continue sautéing for 3 more minutes.

2 Add 2 cups of hot water to the pot or enough to just cover the zucchini (the amount of water may vary depending on the size of the pot). Cover, reduce the heat to low, and simmer for 10 minutes.

3 Add the pasta to the pot, stir, then add 2 more cups of hot water. Continue simmering, stirring occasionally, until the pasta is cooked and the mixture has thickened, about 12 minutes. (If the pasta appears to be dry or undercooked, add small amounts of hot water to the pot to ensure the pasta is covered in the water.). When the pasta is cooked, remove the pot from the heat. Add 2 tablespoons of the grated Parmesan and stir.

4 Divide the pasta into three servings and then top each with 1 ounce of the grated or shaved Parmesan. Sprinkle the remaining sea salt and black pepper over the top of each serving. Store covered in the refrigerator for up to 3 days.

 TIP
If you prefer an even chunkier pasta, you can add more zucchini to the recipe.

EACH SERVING HAS:

Calories **695** • Total fat **29g** • Saturated fat **6g** • Carbohydrate **84g** • Fiber **7g** • Protein **24g**

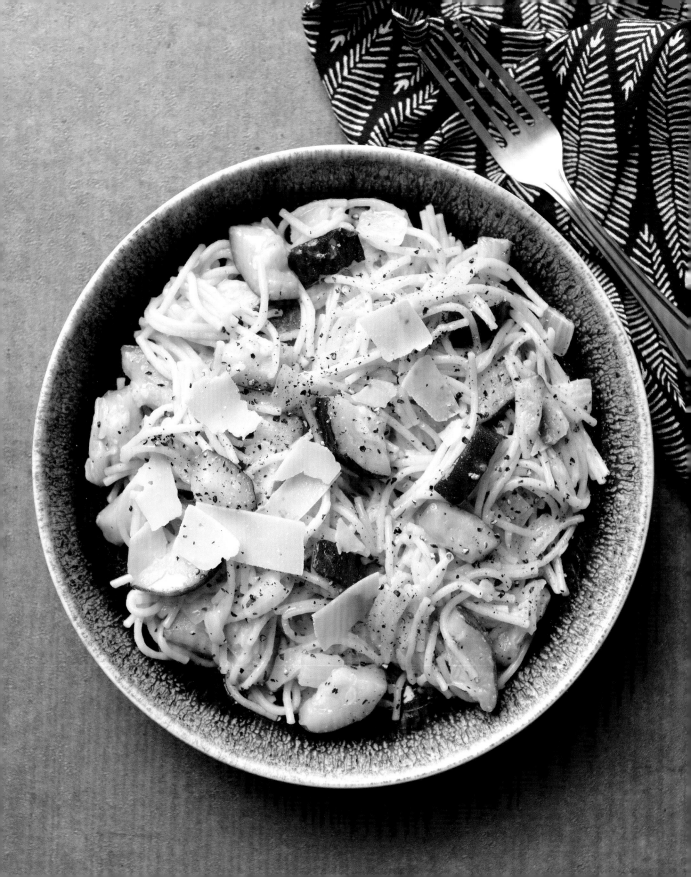

Inspired by a traditional Greek salad, this light and flavorful pasta salad is full of fresh vegetables, capers, olives, and feta. A perfect lunch to bring to work or a picnic, it can be enjoyed warm or cold.

MEDiTERRANEAN PASTA SALAD

4 SERVINGS   **5 MINUTES**   **10 MINUTES**   **1 CUP**

1 cup uncooked whole-grain pasta (rotini or penne)

1 cup cherry tomatoes, halved

1 small cucumber, peeled and chopped into ½-inch (1.25cm) pieces

8 Kalamata olives, pitted and sliced

2 tbsp capers

¼ cup extra virgin olive oil

2 tbsp red wine vinegar

1 tbsp dried oregano

2oz (55g) crumbled feta

1 | Cook the pasta according to package instructions and drain.

2 | In a large bowl, combine the cooked pasta, tomatoes, cucumber, olives, and capers. Mix gently.

3 | In a small bowl, combine the olive oil and vinegar. Whisk with a fork until the ingredients start to thicken.

4 | Add the dressing to the bowl with the pasta and vegetables. Sprinkle the oregano over the top, and gently toss to combine.

5 | Sprinkle the feta over the top, gently toss again, then serve. Store covered in the refrigerator for up to 3 days.

TIP
Salt is not needed for this recipe as the olives, capers, and feta already contain ample salt.

EACH SERVING HAS:

Calories **250** • Total fat **19g** • Saturated fat **4g** • Carbohydrate **15g** • Fiber **3g** • Protein **5g**

This hearty recipe has sweet and salty elements. The eggplant sweetens as it's cooked and, along with the raisins, provides a complex flavor profile to this comforting dish.

PILAF
WiTH EGGPLANT AND RAISINS

 4 SERVINGS   **10 MINUTES**   **30 MINUTES**   **1½ CUPS**

4 eggplant (preferably thinner, about 6oz/170g each) cut into ¼-inch (.5cm) thick slices (if the slices are too large, cut them in half)

1½ tsp fine sea salt, divided

½ cup extra virgin olive oil

1 medium onion (any variety), diced

4 garlic cloves, thinly sliced

¼ cup white wine

1 cup uncooked medium-grain rice

1 (15oz/425g) can crushed tomatoes

3 cups hot water

4 tbsp black raisins

4 tsp finely chopped fresh parsley

4 tsp finely chopped fresh mint

¼ tsp freshly ground black pepper to serve

1 Place the eggplant in a colander and sprinkle with ½ teaspoon of the sea salt. Set aside to rest for 10 minutes, then rinse well and squeeze to remove any remaining water.

2 Add the olive oil to a medium pot placed over medium heat. When the oil begins to shimmer, add the eggplant and sauté for 7 minutes or until soft, moving the eggplant continuously, then add the onions and continue sautéing and stirring for 2 more minutes.

3 Add the garlic and sauté for 1 additional minute, then add the white wine and deglaze the pan. After about 1 minute, add the rice and stir until the rice is coated with the oil.

4 Add the crushed tomatoes, hot water, and remaining sea salt. Stir and bring to a boil, then reduce the heat to low and simmer for 20 minutes. Add more hot water, ¼ cup at a time, if the water level gets too low.

5 Add the raisins, stir, then cover the pot and remove from the heat. Set aside to cool for 15 minutes.

6 To serve, sprinkle 1 teaspoon of the mint and 1 teaspoon of the parsley over each serving, then season each serving with black pepper. Store covered in the refrigerator for up to 3 days.

 TIP

Eggplant can absorb olive oil quite quickly, so make sure you are constantly moving it in the pot while sautéing.

EACH SERVING HAS:

Calories **548** • Total fat **28g** • Saturated fat **4g** • Carbohydrate **67g** • Fiber **9g** • Protein **7g**

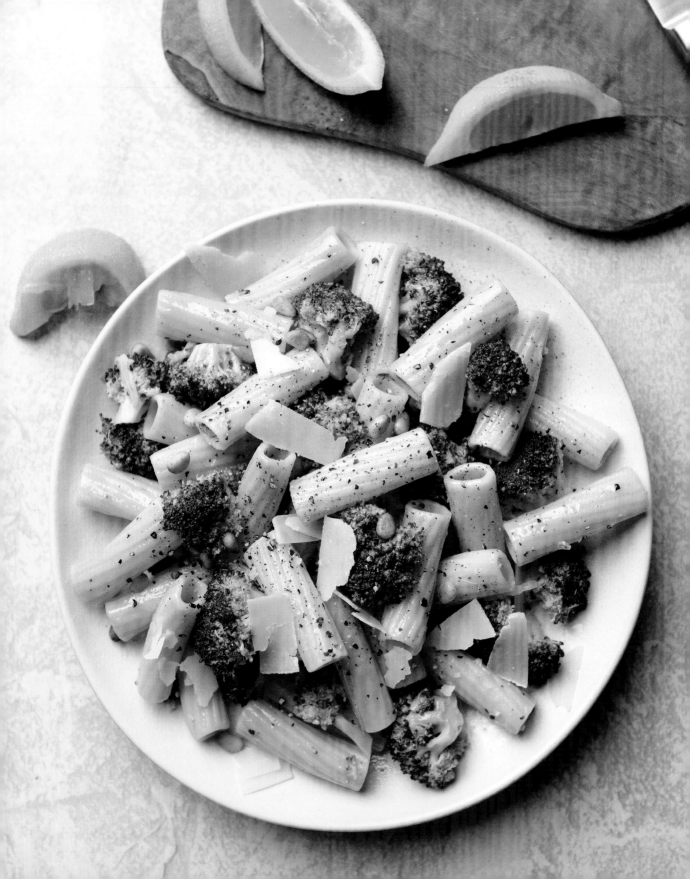

Inspired by a traditional Puglian dish, this recipe transforms broccoli into a delicious, savory sauce, while garlic and anchovies provide an umami flavor.

PUGLIA-STYLE PASTA
WITH BROCCOLI SAUCE

 3 SERVINGS   **15 MINUTES**   **25 MINUTES**   **1½ CUPS**

1lb (450g) fresh broccoli, washed and cut into small florets

7oz (200g) uncooked rigatoni pasta

2 tbsp extra virgin olive oil, plus 1½ tbsp for serving

3 garlic cloves, thinly sliced

2 tbsp pine nuts

4 canned packed-in-oil anchovies

½ tsp kosher salt

3 tsp fresh lemon juice

3oz (85g) grated or shaved Parmesan cheese, divided

½ tsp freshly ground black pepper

1 Place the broccoli in a large pot filled with enough water to cover the broccoli. Bring the pot to a boil and cook for 12 minutes or until the stems can be easily pierced with a fork. Use a slotted spoon to transfer the broccoli to a plate, but do not discard the cooking water. Set the broccoli aside.

2 Add the pasta to the pot with the broccoli water and cook according to package instructions.

3 About 3 minutes before the pasta is ready, place a large, deep pan over medium heat and add 2 tablespoons of the olive oil. When the olive oil is shimmering, add the garlic and sauté for 1 minute, stirring continuously, until the garlic is golden, then add the pine nuts and continue sautéing for 1 more minute.

4 Stir in the anchovies, using a wooden spoon to break them into smaller pieces, then add the broccoli. Continue cooking for 1 additional minute, stirring continuously and using the spoon to break the broccoli into smaller pieces.

5 When the pasta is ready, remove the pot from the heat and drain, reserving ¼ cup of the cooking water.

6 Add the pasta and 2 tablespoons of the cooking water to the pan, stirring until all the ingredients are well combined. Cook for 1 minute, then remove the pan from the heat.

7 Promptly divide the pasta among three plates. Top each serving with a pinch of kosher salt, 1 teaspoon of the lemon juice, 1 ounce of the Parmesan, 1½ teaspoons of the remaining olive oil, and a pinch of fresh ground pepper. Store covered in the refrigerator for up to 3 days.

EACH SERVING HAS:

Calories **499** • Total fat **21g** • Saturated fat **3g** • Carbohydrate **61g** • Fiber **6g** • Protein **17g**

Filled with sweet leeks and tangy feta wrapped in a flaky phyllo crust, this traditional Greek savory pie is great as an appetizer, snack, or main course.

LEEK AND FETA PIE

 6 SERVINGS   **10 MINUTES**   **1 HOUR 5 MINUTES**   **1 PIECE**

¼ cup extra virgin olive oil plus ⅓ cup for brushing

3 spring onions (white parts only), cut into ½-inch (1.25cm) slices

4 cups sliced leeks (white ends only), cut into ½-inch (1.25cm) slices

12 (14 x 18-in/35.5 x 46cm) phyllo sheets, defrosted

¼ tsp fine sea salt

¼ tsp freshly ground black pepper

¼ cup chopped fresh dill

4oz (115g) finely crumbled feta

2 eggs, beaten

1½ tbsp unseasoned breadcrumbs

1 Preheat the oven at 350°F (180°C) and brush a 10-inch round baking pan with olive oil.

2 Add ¼ cup of the olive oil to a large pan over medium heat. When the oil begins to shimmer, add the spring onions and sauté for about 5 minutes or until the onions are soft, then add the leeks and continue sautéing, stirring continuously, until the leeks soften and there is no liquid left in the pan, about 15–20 minutes. Transfer the contents of the pan to a large bowl and set aside to cool.

3 Prepare the crust by placing the first phyllo sheet in the base of the prepared baking pan, ensuring the edges of the sheet hang over the edges of the pan. Brush the sheet with olive oil, then place another phyllo sheet crosswise in the pan and brush it with olive oil. Continue until you have 6 phyllo sheets layered one on top of the other.

4 Add the sea salt, black pepper, dill, and feta to the cooled leek mixture and mix well, then add the eggs, mix, then add the breadcrumbs and mix again. Empty the filling into the pan with the phyllo, using a spatula to evenly spread the mixture over the dough sheets. Trim the edges of the sheets, leaving about an inch hanging over the edge of pan, then fold the remaining edge in and over the top of the filling.

5 Make the top crust by layering and brushing the remaining phyllo sheets over the top of the pie. Trim the edges of the hanging phyllo sheets, leaving about 1 inch (2.5cm), and then twist the edges around the pan to form a border. Brush the border with the remaining olive oil.

6 Use a sharp knife to score the pie into 6 equal-sized pieces, but do not cut all the way through. Sprinkle a few drops of water over the pie and then place it in the oven for 40 minutes or until the phyllo is golden.

7 Remove the pie from the oven and set it aside to cool for at least 15 minutes before cutting into 6 equal-sized pieces. Serve warm or at room temperature. Store covered in the refrigerator for up to 3 days. (Bring to room temperature before serving.)

EACH SERVING HAS:

Calories **418**   •   Total fat **29g**   •   Saturated fat **7g**   •   Carbohydrate **31g**   •   Fiber **2g**   •   Protein **8g**

This delicious and easy pasta dish combines all the quintessential Mediterranean ingredients: tomatoes, olives, capers, garlic, and anchovies.

SPAGHETTi ALLA PUTTANESCA

 4 SERVINGS   **5 MINUTES**   **25 MINUTES**   **1¼ CUPS**

¼ cup extra virgin olive oil

2 garlic cloves

1 small dried chili pepper (any variety), sliced

3oz (85g) canned anchovies, rinsed and drained

14oz (395g) chopped fresh tomatoes or canned crushed tomatoes

¼ cup whole Kalamata olives, sliced

¼ cup capers, rinsed and chopped

2 tbsp chopped fresh parsley

¼ tsp fine sea salt

½lb (225g) uncooked spaghetti

Freshly ground black pepper, for serving

1 Fill a large pot with cold water and place it over high heat.

2 Add the olive oil to a medium pan placed over medium heat. When the oil begins to shimmer, add the garlic cloves and chili pepper. Sauté until the cloves begin to brown, then add the anchovies and sauté for 3–5 minutes, mashing the anchovies with a fork or spatula.

3 Add the tomatoes, olives, capers, parsley, and sea salt. Reduce the heat to medium-low and simmer for 10 minutes.

4 While the sauce is simmering, place the pasta in the boiling water and reduce the heat to medium. Cook according to instructions, then drain and return the cooked pasta to the pot.

5 Add the sauce to the pot with the pasta and stir to combine. Heat for 1–2 minutes, then transfer the pasta and sauce to a platter and season with the black pepper. Serve promptly. Store covered in the refrigerator for up to 3 days.

 TIP
You can make the sauce ahead of time and store it in the refrigerator for up to 2 days. When you're ready to use it, reheat the sauce in a pan placed over low heat.

EACH SERVING HAS:

Calories **454** • Total fat **21g** • Saturated fat **3g** • Carbohydrate **50g** • Fiber **4g** • Protein **15g**

This classic Greek savory pie is made with spinach, feta, and herbs, and is surrounded by flaky phyllo dough. Frozen spinach is used to make this impressive dish easy to prepare.

SPANAKOPITA
(GREEK SPINACH PIE)

 8 SERVINGS   10 MINUTES   50 MINUTES   1 PIECE

1lb (455g) frozen spinach, thawed and drained

2 tbsp extra virgin olive oil plus ¼ cup for brushing

1 medium onion (any variety), diced

3 tbsp chopped fresh parsley

2 tbsp chopped fresh dill

¼ cup chopped fresh mint

¼ tsp ground nutmeg

½ tsp granulated sugar

10oz (285g) feta

3 eggs, beaten

¼ tsp freshly ground black pepper

12 (14 x 18-in/35.5 x 46cm) phyllo sheets, defrosted

1 Preheat the oven to 350°F (180°C). Squeeze the spinach to remove as much of the moisture as possible.

2 Heat 2 tablespoons of the olive oil in a medium pan over medium heat. Once the oil is shimmering, add the onions and sauté until soft, about 6 minutes. Add the spinach and sauté for 2 more minutes, then remove the pan from the heat and empty the mixture into a large bowl. Add the parsley, dill, mint, nutmeg, and sugar. Mix well and then set aside to cool for 10 minutes.

3 Grate half of the feta using the largest holes of a box grater and then crumble the other half. In a medium bowl, combine the eggs, feta, and black pepper. Mix well, then add the egg mixture to the spinach mixture and stir until the ingredients are well combined.

4 Brush a 10 x 15-inch (25 x 40cm) pan with olive oil, then place a sheet of the phyllo dough in the pan and brush with the olive oil. Repeat the process with 5 more phyllo sheets, brushing each sheet with olive oil before layering in the next sheet. Spread the spinach mixture evenly over the bottom crust.

5 Make the top crust by covering the spinach mixture with 5–6 phyllo sheets, brushing each sheet with olive oil and then trimming away any phyllo hanging over the edge of the pan or simply rolling it up into a crust.

6 Use a sharp knife to score the top of the pie into 8 equal-sized pieces, but do not cut all the way through the dough sheets. Sprinkle the top crust with a few drops of water.

7 Bake for 35–40 minutes or until the phyllo turns golden brown. Lift one side of the pie to ensure the bottom is completely baked, then remove the pie from the oven and set aside to cool for 1 hour before cutting into pieces. Store in an airtight container in the refrigerator for up to 3 days.

EACH SERVING HAS:

Calories **315** • Total fat **21g** • Saturated fat **8g** • Carbohydrate **20g** • Fiber **2g** • Protein **11g**

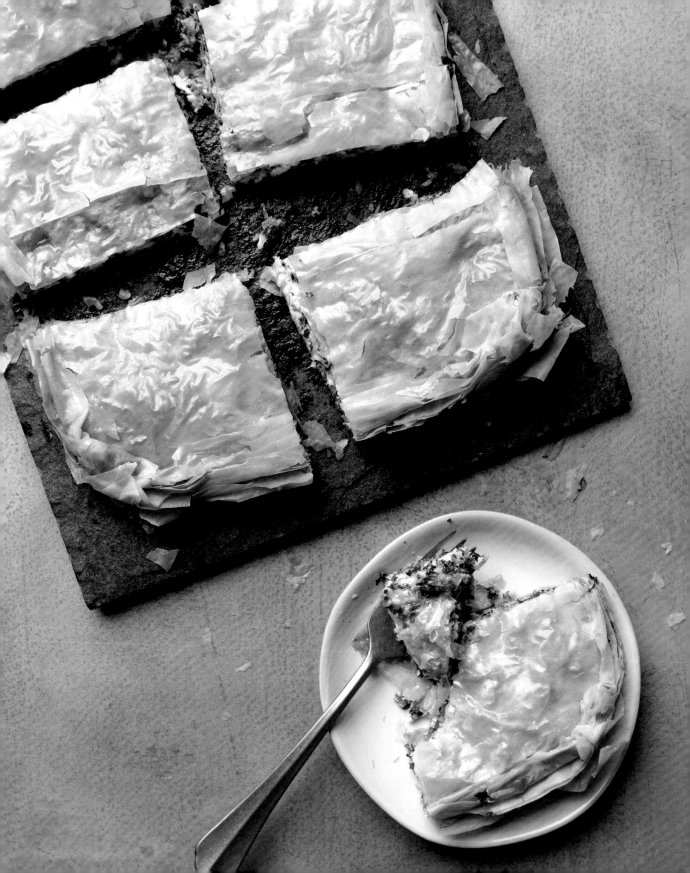

This comforting rice dish is made with only the simplest ingredients—tomatoes, onions, and olive oil—and then cooked until soft and creamy. It's perfect as a main dish when accompanied by a simple green salad.

ToMATo R!CE

 3 SERVINGS  **10 MINUTES**   **25 MINUTES** **1¼ CUPS**

2 tbsp extra virgin olive oil

1 medium onion (any variety), chopped

1 garlic clove, finely chopped

1 cup uncooked medium-grain rice

1 tbsp tomato paste

1lb (450g) canned crushed tomatoes, or 1lb (450g) fresh tomatoes (puréed in a food processor)

¾ tsp fine sea salt

1 tsp granulated sugar

2 cups hot water

2 tbsp chopped fresh mint or basil

1 Heat the olive oil in a wide, deep pan over medium heat. When the oil begins to shimmer, add the onion and sauté for 3–4 minutes or until soft, then add the garlic and sauté for an additional 30 seconds.

2 Add the rice and stir until the rice is coated with the oil, then add the tomato paste and stir rapidly. Add the tomatoes, sea salt, and sugar, and then stir again.

3 Add the hot water, stir, then reduce the heat to low and simmer, covered, for 20 minutes or until the rice is soft. (If the rice appears to need more cooking time, add a small amount of hot water to the pan and continue cooking.) Remove the pan from the heat.

4 Add the chopped mint or basil, and let the rice sit for 10 minutes before serving. Store covered in the refrigerator for up to 4 days.

 TIP
A dollop of Greek yogurt adds a hint of tanginess that pairs well with the rice.

EACH SERVING HAS:
Calories **384** • Total fat **10g** • Saturated fat **1g** • Carbohydrate **67g** • Fiber **5g** • Protein **7g**

This orzo salad is full of flavor, with balsamic-marinated peppers that are paired perfectly with tangy, peppery feta cheese. It's an ideal salad for a work lunch or a picnic.

ORZO
WITH FETA AND MARINATED PEPPERS

 2 SERVINGS   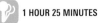 **1 HOUR 25 MINUTES**   **37 MINUTES**   **1½ CUPS**

2 medium red bell peppers

¼ cup extra virgin olive oil

1 tbsp balsamic vinegar plus 1 tsp for serving

¼ tsp ground cumin

Pinch of ground cinnamon

Pinch of ground cloves

¼ tsp fine sea salt plus a pinch for the orzo

1 cup uncooked orzo

3oz (85g) crumbled feta

1 tbsp chopped fresh basil

¼ tsp freshly ground black pepper

1 Preheat the oven at 350°F (180°C). Place the peppers on a baking pan and roast in the oven for 25 minutes or until they're soft and can be pierced with a fork. Set aside to cool for 10 minutes.

2 While the peppers are roasting, combine the olive oil, 1 tablespoon of the balsamic vinegar, cumin, cinnamon, cloves, and ¼ teaspoon of the sea salt. Stir to combine, then set aside.

3 Peel the cooled peppers, remove the seeds, and then chop into large pieces. Place the peppers in the olive oil and vinegar mixture and then toss to coat, ensuring the peppers are covered in the marinade. Cover and place in the refrigerator to marinate for 20 minutes.

4 While the peppers are marinating, prepare the orzo by bringing 3 cups of water and a pinch of salt to a boil in a large pot over high heat. When the water is boiling, add the orzo, reduce the heat to medium, and cook, stirring occasionally, for 10–12 minutes or until soft, then drain and transfer to a serving bowl.

5 Add the peppers and marinade to the orzo, mixing well, then place in the refrigerator and to cool for at least 1 hour.

6 To serve, top with the feta, basil, black pepper, and 1 teaspoon of the balsamic vinegar. Mix well, and serve promptly. Store covered in the refrigerator for up to 3 days.

 TIP

This is an ideal make-ahead recipe. You can prepare the marinated peppers and orzo up to 2 days ahead and store in the refrigerator until ready to serve.

EACH SERVING HAS:

Calories **392** • Total fat **36g** • Saturated fat **10g** • Carbohydrate **9g** • Fiber **3g** • Protein **7g**

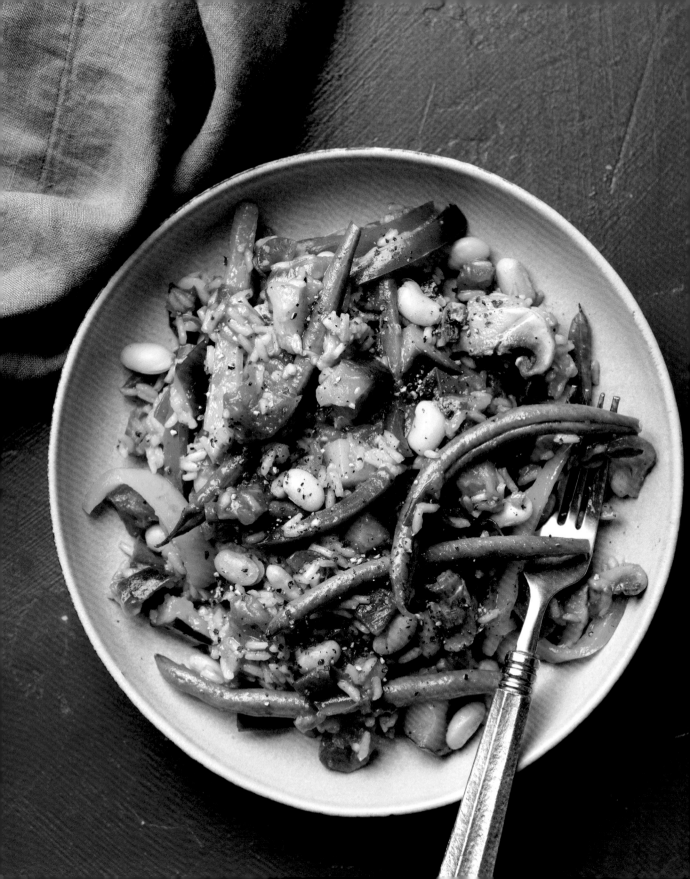

This aromatic vegetarian paella is loaded with vegetables, flavor, and color. The mushrooms and eggplant provide both texture and satiety.

VEGETARIAN PAELLA

 6 SERVINGS   **10 MINUTES**    **35 MINUTES**   **1½ CUPS**

½ tsp saffron threads

3 tbsp warm water

6 tbsp extra virgin olive oil

1 medium red onion, sliced

1 medium red bell pepper, seeded and sliced

1 medium yellow bell pepper, seeded and sliced

1 medium Italian eggplant, cubed

3 garlic cloves, minced

1 cup uncooked medium-grain rice

2 cups vegetable broth

3 medium ripe tomatoes (any variety), chopped, or 1 (15oz/425g) can chopped tomatoes

½ tsp smoked paprika

¼ tsp freshly ground black pepper

1½ tsp fine sea salt

4oz (115g) white button mushrooms, sliced

4oz (115g) green beans (fresh or frozen)

1 (15oz /425g) can white beans

1 In a small bowl, combine the saffron threads and warm water. Set aside to steep.

2 Add the olive oil to a large, deep pan over medium heat. When the oil is shimmering, add the onions and sauté for 2–3 minutes or until soft, then add the bell peppers and eggplant and sauté for 5 more minutes, stirring frequently.

3 Add the garlic and continue sautéing for 1 more minute, stirring constantly, then add the rice and stir continuously for 1 minute until the rice is completely coated in the oil.

4 Add the vegetable broth, tomatoes, saffron threads with steeping water, smoked paprika, black pepper, and sea salt.

5 Bring the mixture to a boil, then reduce the heat to low and simmer for 15 minutes, stirring occasionally. (If the rice becomes too dry while cooking, add 1–2 tablespoons of hot water and stir.)

6 Add the mushrooms, green beans, and white beans, and mix gently. Continue cooking for 10 more minutes, then remove the pan from the heat and serve promptly. Store covered in the refrigerator for up to 3 days.

 TIP
If you are using a ready-made broth that contains salt, omit the salt in the recipe.

EACH SERVING HAS:

Calories **376** • Total fat **14g** • Saturated fat **2g** • Carbohydrate **52g** • Fiber **7g** • Protein **10g**

CHAPTER FIVE

SEAFOOD, MEAT, AND POULTRY ENTRÉES

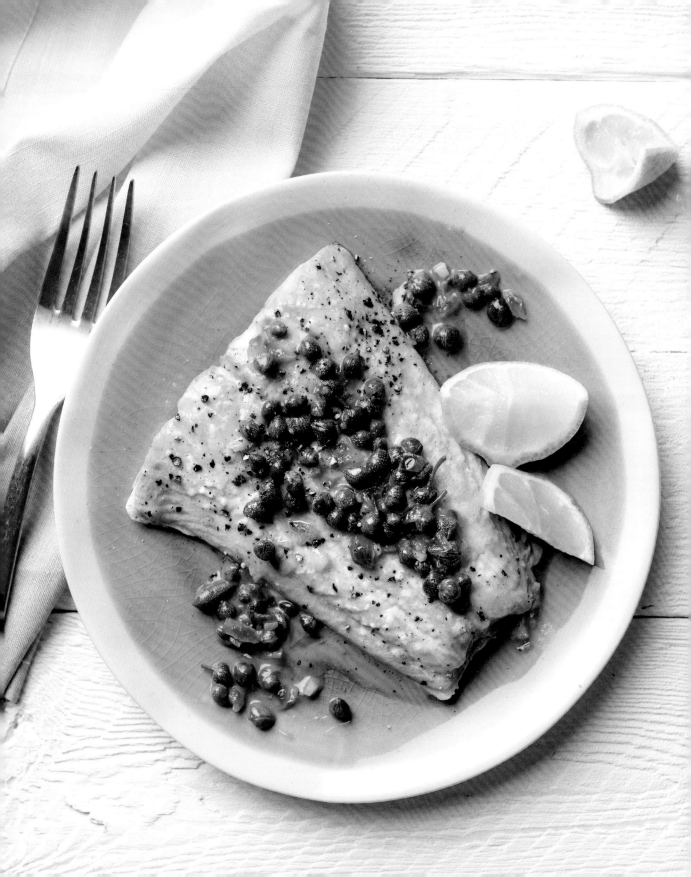

A lemon caper sauce provides a burst of citrusy flavor to this roasted salmon, which goes perfectly when paired with boiled greens or a tossed salad.

CiTRUS MEDiTERRANEAN SALMON
WiTH LEMON CAPER SAUCE

 2 SERVINGS   **15 MINUTES**   **22 MINUTES**   **1 FILLET AND 1½ TBSP SAUCE**

2 tbsp fresh lemon juice

⅓ cup orange juice

1 tbsp extra virgin olive oil

⅛ tsp freshly ground black pepper

2 (6oz/170g) salmon fillets

For the lemon caper sauce

2 tbsp extra virgin olive oil

1 tbsp finely chopped red onion

1 garlic clove, minced

2 tbsp fresh lemon juice

5fl oz (150ml) dry white wine

2 tbsp capers, rinsed

⅛ tsp freshly ground black pepper

1 | Preheat the oven to 350°F (180°C).

2 | In a small bowl, combine the lemon juice, orange juice, olive oil, and black pepper. Whisk until blended, then pour the mixture into a zipper-lock bag. Place the fillets in the bag, shake gently, and transfer the salmon to the refrigerator to marinate for 10 minutes.

3 | When the salmon is done marinating, transfer the fillets and marinade to a medium baking dish. Bake for 10–15 minutes or until the salmon is cooked through and the internal temperature reaches 165°F (75°C). Remove the salmon from the oven and cover loosely with foil. Set aside to rest.

4 | While the salmon is resting, make the lemon caper sauce by heating the olive oil in a medium pan over medium heat. When the olive oil begins to shimmer, add the onions and sauté for 3 minutes, stirring frequently, then add the garlic and sauté for another 30 seconds.

5 | Add the lemon juice and wine. Bring the mixture to a boil and cook until the sauce becomes thick, about 2–3 minutes, then remove the pan from the heat. Add the capers and black pepper, and stir.

6 | Transfer the fillets to 2 plates, and spoon 1½ tablespoons of the sauce over each fillet. Store covered in the refrigerator for up to 3 days.

EACH SERVING HAS:

Calories **414** • Total fat **28g** • Saturated fat **4g** • Carbohydrate **10g** • Fiber **1g** • Protein **32g**

This simply delicious fish is baked until crispy and coated with an garlic-herb seasoning. It features a crunchy topping on the outside and tender, flaky fish on the inside.

MEDITERRANEAN GARLIC AND HERB-ROASTED COD

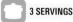 3 SERVINGS   10 MINUTES   15 MINUTES   1 FILLET

4½ tbsp extra virgin olive oil plus 1 tsp for brushing

1½ tbsp dried oregano

1 tsp paprika

1½ tsp dried onion flakes

½ tsp salt

¼ tsp freshly ground black pepper

1½ tbsp fresh lemon juice plus extra for serving

1 garlic clove, minced

3 tsp Dijon mustard

1lb (450g) cod fillets (about 3–4), patted dry

2 tbsp chopped fresh parsley

For the topping

1½ tbsp extra virgin olive oil

4 tbsp unseasoned breadcrumbs

1 Preheat the oven to 430°F (220°C). Brush a baking dish large enough to hold the fish in a single layer with 1 teaspoon of the olive oil.

2 In a small bowl, combine the oregano, paprika, onion flakes, salt, and black pepper. Mix well and set aside.

3 In a medium bowl, combine 4½ tablespoons of the olive oil, lemon juice, garlic, and Dijon mustard. Add the dry ingredients to the wet ingredients and mix well.

4 Dip each fillet in the coating and toss to coat, then place the fillets in the dish and drizzle the leftover coating over the top of the fillets.

5 Make the breadcrumb topping by combining the breadcrumbs and olive oil in a small bowl and mixing with a fork. Sprinkle the breadcrumb mixture over the fillets.

6 Place in the oven and roast for 15 minutes or until the breadcrumb topping becomes golden brown.

7 Transfer to a plate and top with the chopped parsley and a squeeze of lemon. (This recipe is best eaten fresh.)

EACH SERVING HAS:

Calories **403** • Total fat **29g** • Saturated fat **4g** • Carbohydrate **11g** • Fiber **1g** • Protein **24g**

This traditional Greek preparation features roasted fish in a rich tomato and onion sauce with a light and crunchy crust. Serve over a dressed green salad or sautéed spinach.

PSARI A LA SPETSIOTA
(OVEN-ROASTED FISH WITH TOMATO AND ONION)

 3 SERVINGS   **1 HOUR 10 MINUTES**   **50 MINUTES**   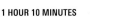 **1¼ FILLETS**

4 medium sea bream, snapper, or other white meat fish fillets (about 1lb/455g)

¼ tsp salt

Juice of 1 lemon

⅓ cup extra virgin olive oil plus 3 tsp for the breadcrumbs and drizzling

1 medium onion (any variety), chopped

3 garlic cloves, finely chopped

⅓ cup white cooking wine

3 medium tomatoes, chopped, or 18oz (510g) canned chopped tomatoes

½ cup chopped fresh parsley, divided

½ tsp freshly ground black pepper

¼ cup unseasoned breadcrumbs

1 Place the fillets in a shallow baking dish. Sprinkle the salt over the top of the fillets, then drizzle the lemon juice over the top. Cover the dish with plastic wrap and transfer to the refrigerator to marinate for 1 hour. When the marinating time is complete, remove the fish from the refrigerator and preheat the oven to 350°F (175°C).

2 Place a medium pan over medium heat and add the olive oil. When the oil is shimmering, add the onions and sauté until soft, then add the garlic and sauté for 1 more minute.

3 Add the wine to the pan and let the mixture simmer until the liquid has evaporated, then add the tomatoes, ¼ cup of the parsley, and the black pepper. Let the sauce simmer for an additional 20 minutes.

4 Once the sauce is ready, spread 3 tablespoons across the bottom of a medium baking dish. Place the fish fillets on top of the sauce, ensuring the fillets fit snuggly in the dish.

5 Spread the remaining sauce over the top of the fish, ensuring the fish is completely covered with the sauce. Set aside.

6 Combine the breadcrumbs, 2 teaspoons of the olive oil, and the remaining ¼ cup parsley in a small bowl. Use a fork to mix the ingredients, then sprinkle the breadcrumb mixture over the fish. Transfer to the oven and bake for 30 minutes.

7 Transfer the fish to a plate and top with the sauce from the baking dish. Drizzle the remaining teaspoon of olive oil over the fish before serving. Store in an airtight container in the refrigerator for up to 3 days.

EACH SERVING HAS:

Calories **476** • Total fat **31g** • Saturated fat **4g** • Carbohydrate **17g** • Fiber **3g** • Protein **33g**

This shrimp is cooked in a flavorful tomato sauce with a splash of ouzo, topped with crumbled feta, and then finished in the oven. Serve on a bed of rice as a main course or in smaller amounts as an appetizer.

SHRIMP AND FETA SAGANAKI

 2 SERVINGS   **10 MINUTES**   **35 MINUTES**   🍴 **10 SHRIMP**

1¼lb (565g) raw medium shrimp (about 20), peeled and deveined

¼ tsp fine sea salt

¼ tsp freshly ground black pepper

4 tbsp extra virgin olive oil, divided

5 garlic cloves, minced

¼ cup ouzo (anise-flavored liquor)

½ large onion (any variety), chopped

1 small hot chili, sliced

1 tsp red pepper flakes

14oz (400g) canned crushed tomatoes or whole tomatoes chopped in a food processor

1 tsp dried oregano, divided

3oz (85g) crumbled feta, divided

1 tbsp chopped fresh basil

1 Preheat the oven to 400°F (200°C). Pat the shrimp dry with paper towels, then season with the sea salt and black pepper.

2 Add 2 tablespoons of the olive oil to a large skillet over medium-high heat. When the oil begins to shimmer, add the shrimp and sauté for about 2 minutes and then add the garlic and sauté for 1 more minute or until the shrimp turn pink.

3 Add the ouzo and sauté for 2 minutes or until the alcohol has evaporated. Remove the pan from the heat and set aside.

4 Add the remaining 2 tablespoons of olive oil to a medium pot or saucepan placed over medium heat. When the olive oil begins to shimmer, add the onions and sauté for 5 minutes or until translucent. Add the sliced chili and red pepper flakes and sauté for 2 more minutes. Add the tomatoes, cover, and simmer for 7 minutes or until the sauce thickens.

5 Pour the tomato sauce into an oven-proof casserole dish or cast-iron skillet large enough to hold the shrimp in a single layer. Sprinkle ½ teaspoon of the oregano and half of the feta over the sauce, then place the shrimp on top of the sauce, lightly pressing each shrimp into the sauce. Sprinkle the remaining feta and oregano over the shrimp.

6 Transfer to the oven and bake for 15 minutes, then top with the chopped basil. Store covered in the refrigerator for up to 2 days.

 TIP
You may replace the ouzo with an equal amount of white wine.

EACH SERVING HAS:

Calories **659** • Total fat **40g** • Saturated fat **11g** • Carbohydrate **27g** • Fiber **5g** • Protein **49g**

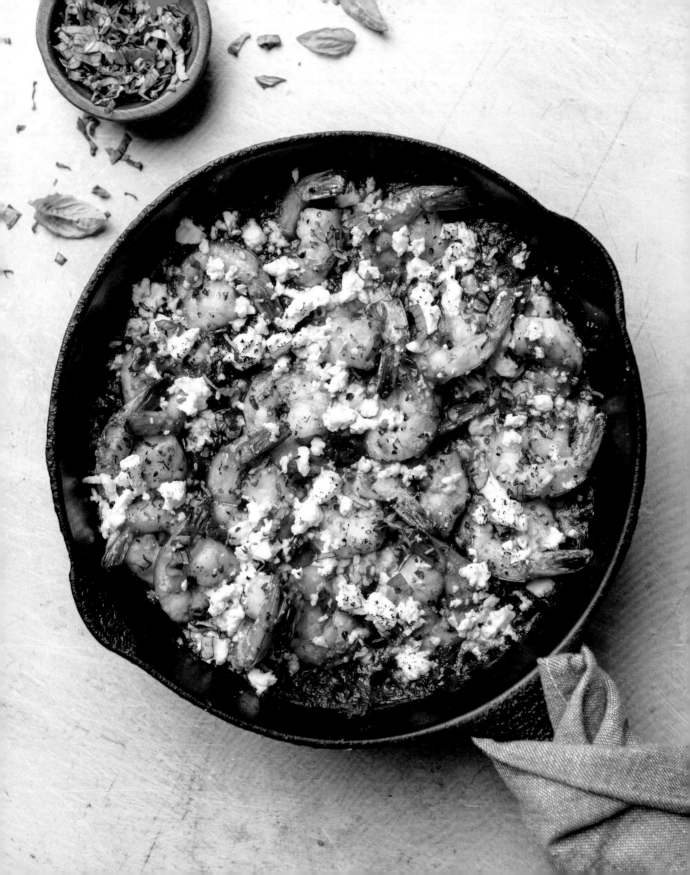

A classic combination: succulent shrimp sautéed with a garlic, lemon, and olive oil sauce. Serve with pasta or rice and vegetables for a complete meal, or as a meze or tapas dish accompanied by some white wine.

SAUTÉED GARLIC-LEMON SHRIMP

 3 SERVINGS   5 MINUTES   5 MINUTES   7 SHRIMP

1¼lb (565g) uncooked medium shrimp (about 20), peeled and deveined

⅓ cup extra virgin olive oil, divided

5 garlic cloves, minced

2 tbsp fresh lemon juice

Zest of 1 lemon

¼ cup ouzo (anise-flavored liquor)

2 tbsp chopped fresh parsley

¼ tsp fine sea salt

A pinch of freshly ground black pepper

1 Pat the shrimp dry with paper towels. Add 3 tablespoons of the olive oil to a large pan over medium heat. When the oil is shimmering, add the shrimp and sauté for about 2 minutes, then add the garlic and continue sautéing until the garlic becomes fragrant, about 30 seconds.

2 Add the lemon juice, lemon zest, ouzo, and parsley. Cook for 2 minutes or until the shrimp is cooked through and develops a uniform pink color, and then remove the shrimp from the heat.

3 Sprinkle the sea salt and black pepper over the top of the shrimp, then drizzle the remaining olive oil over the shrimp. Serve promptly.

 TIP
If desired, you can substitute an equal amount of white wine for the ouzo.

EACH SERVING HAS:
Calories **345** • Total fat **26g** • Saturated fat **4g** • Carbohydrate **3g** • Fiber **0g** • Protein **26g**

This tender and juicy chicken breast is marinated in lemon and oregano, lightly grilled, and finished in the oven. It's delicious eaten straight off the skewer or added to a salad for a boost of protein.

CHICKEN SOUVLAKI

 4 SERVINGS   **25 MINUTES**   **25 MINUTES**   **2 SKEWERS**

¼ cup extra virgin olive oil plus 1 tsp for brushing the pan

2 tbsp fresh lemon juice plus juice of 1 lemon for serving

1 tbsp dried oregano

1¼lb (565g) boneless, skinless chicken breasts, cut into bite-sized pieces (about 48 pieces)

1 medium green bell pepper, seeded and cut into square pieces no larger than 1 inch (2.5cm)

1 medium red bell pepper, seeded and cut into square pieces no larger than 1 inch (2.5cm)

8 wooden skewers

½ tsp salt

1 Combine the olive oil, 2 tablespoons of the lemon juice, and oregano in a plastic zipper lock bag. Seal the bag tightly and gently shake to combine, then add the chicken pieces and carefully rotate the bag until the chicken is coated in the marinade. Transfer to the refrigerator to rest for at least 15 minutes.

2 Preheat the oven at 350°F (180°C). Remove the chicken from the marinade. Thread the chicken and bell pepper pieces onto the skewers, adding a piece of bell pepper for every 2 pieces of chicken, until there is a total of 6 chicken pieces on each skewer.

3 Lightly brush a grill pan or frying pan with olive oil and then place the pan over medium-high heat.

4 When the pan is hot, place 4 skewers in the pan. Cook for 1 minute and then rotate the skewers halfway and cook for another minute. Transfer the skewers to a large sheet pan and promptly transfer to the preheated oven to bake for 10–12 minutes or until the internal temperature reaches 165°F (75°C).

5 While the first batch of skewers is baking, repeat the browning process with the remaining skewers. When the first batch of skewers is done baking, set aside to cool and then place the next batch in the oven. Repeat until all the skewers are baked.

6 Sprinkle the salt over the skewers and then drizzle the juice of 1 lemon over the top. Store covered in the refrigerator for up to 2 days.

 TIP

This is delicious when served with a sliced tomato, pita bread, and a dollop of Greek yogurt or tzatziki sauce.

EACH SERVING HAS:

Calories **272** • Total fat **16g** • Saturated fat **2g** • Carbohydrate **4g** • Fiber **1g** • Protein **29g**

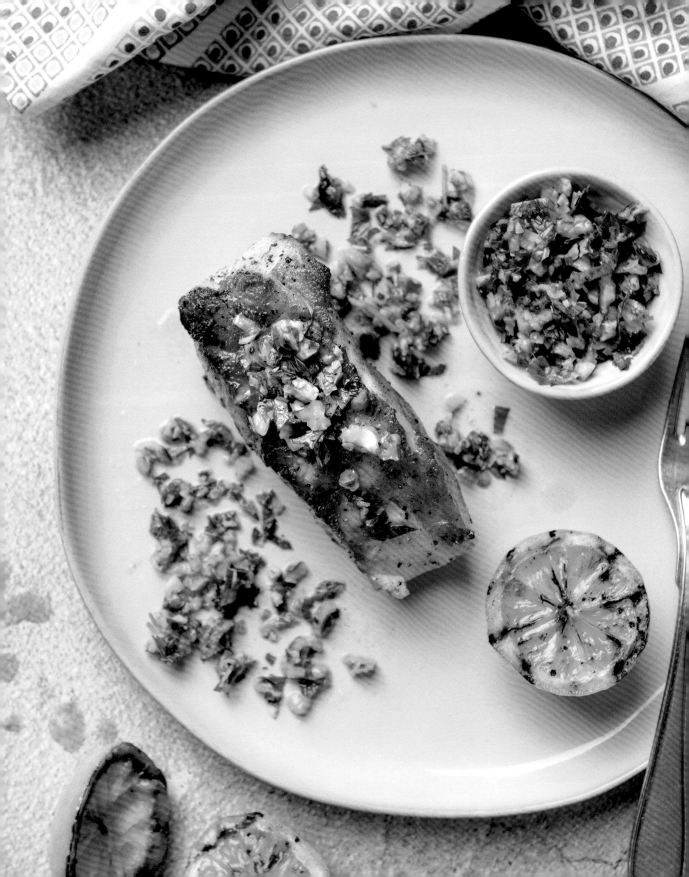

This flavorful, fresh fish is grilled until golden and then topped with gremolata, an Italian sauce made with parsley, lemon zest, garlic, and toasted walnuts.

GRILLED FISH
WITH WALNUT GREMOLATA

 2 SERVINGS　　 **10 MINUTES**　　 **10 MINUTES**　　 **1 FILLET WITH 2 TBSP GREMOLATA**

2 firm white fish fillets, such as sea bass, cod, or grouper (about 1lb/455g)

2 tbsp extra virgin olive oil, divided

1 tsp fine sea salt, divided

1 tsp freshly ground black pepper, divided

Juice of 1 large lemon for serving

For the gremolata

12 walnut halves

¼ cup chopped fresh parsley

Zest of 1 large lemon

1 garlic clove, minced

2 tsp extra virgin olive oil

1 In a small pan over low heat, toast the walnut halves for 2 minutes or until they begin to brown, then promptly remove from the heat and transfer to a small bowl to cool.

2 Finely chop the cooled walnuts and place them in a medium bowl with the parsley, lemon zest, garlic, and olive oil. Mix well, cover, and set aside.

3 Place the fish fillets on a plate. Brush 1 teaspoon of the olive oil over each side and then sprinkle ¼ teaspoon sea salt and ¼ teaspoon black pepper over each fillet.

4 Brush a grill pan with the remaining 2 teaspoons of olive oil and then preheat the pan over high heat for 3 minutes. Lay the fillets on the hot pan and reduce the heat to medium. Grill the fillets for 3–4 minutes, depending on the thickness of the fish, then turn and grill for 3 more minutes or until the fish is golden and has reached an internal temperature of 145°F (65°C). Transfer the fish to a serving platter.

5 Squeeze the lemon over the fillets and then top each fillet with 2 tablespoons of the gremolata. The gremolata can be stored in the refrigerator for up to 2 days. (The fish is best eaten fresh.)

 TIP
If you don't have a grill pan, you can use an outdoor grill, or simply pan-fry the fish using the same method.

EACH SERVING HAS:

Calories **467**　•　Total fat **31g**　•　Saturated fat **5g**　•　Carbohydrate **3g**　•　Fiber **1g**　•　Protein **44g**

This traditional recipe is made with pork that's stewed until tender and paired with plenty of greens. Lemon juice adds brightness and flavor to this hearty and comforting meal.

STEWED PORK
WITH GREENS

 3 SERVINGS

 10 MINUTES

1 HOUR 40 MINUTES

6OZ (170G) PORK AND 1 CUP GREENS

¾ tsp fine sea salt, divided

½ tsp freshly ground black pepper, divided

1¼lb (565g) pork shoulder, trimmed and cut into 1½-inch (3.75cm) chunks

6 tbsp extra virgin olive oil, divided

1 bay leaf

3 allspice berries

2 tbsp dry red wine

1 medium onion (any variety), chopped

2 spring onions, sliced (white parts only)

1 leek, sliced (white parts only)

¼ cup chopped fresh dill

1lb (450g) Swiss chard, roughly chopped

3 tbsp fresh lemon juice plus more for serving

1 Sprinkle ¼ teaspoon of the sea salt and ¼ teaspoon of the black pepper over the pork. Rub the seasonings into the meat.

2 Add 1 tablespoon of the olive oil to a heavy pan over medium-high heat. Add the bay leaf and allspice berries, then add the meat and brown for 2–3 minutes per side.

3 Add the red wine and let it bubble, then use a wooden spatula to scrape the browned bits from the pan. Continue simmering until the liquid has evaporated, about 3 minutes, then transfer the meat and juices to a plate. Set aside.

4 Heat 4 tablespoons of the olive oil in a large pot placed over medium heat. Add the onion, spring onions, and leeks, and sauté until soft, about 5 minutes, then add the dill and sauté for 1–2 minutes more.

5 Add the meat and juices to the pot and sprinkle another ¼ teaspoon sea salt and ¼ teaspoon black pepper over the meat. Add just enough hot water to cover the meat halfway (start with less water), then cover and reduce the heat to low. Simmer for about 1 hour or until the meat is tender.

6 Remove the lid and add the chard and lemon juice. Use tongs to toss the chard and mix well. Continue simmering for about 5 minutes, then drizzle in the last tablespoon of olive oil and mix again. Cover and simmer for another 20 minutes, mixing occasionally, until the greens are wilted, then remove the pot from the heat.

7 Let stand covered for 10 minutes, then add a squeeze of lemon before serving. Allow to cool completely before covering and storing in the refrigerator for up to 2 days.

EACH SERVING HAS:

Calories **609** • Total fat **41g** • Saturated fat **9g** • Carbohydrate **17g** • Fiber **7g** • Protein **43g**

This classic Greek comfort food features tender beef stewed with spices and tomato. Serve with a green leafy salad and good hearty bread, or with your favorite pasta.

HEARTY STEWED BEEF IN ToMATo SAUCE

 5 SERVINGS

 20 MINUTES

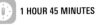 1 HOUR 45 MINUTES

2 PIECES WITH SAUCE

3 tbsp extra virgin olive oil

2lb (905g) boneless beef chuck, cut into 2-inch (5cm) chunks

1 medium onion (any variety), diced

4 garlic cloves, minced

⅓ cup white wine

2 tbsp tomato paste

1 cinnamon stick

4 cloves

4 allspice berries

1 bay leaf

¼ tsp freshly ground black pepper

15oz (425g) canned crushed tomatoes or chopped fresh tomatoes

1 cup hot water

½ tsp fine sea salt

1 Add the olive oil to a deep pan over medium heat. When the oil starts to shimmer, place half the beef in the pan. Brown the meat until a crust develops, about 3–4 minutes per side, then transfer the meat to a plate, and set aside. Repeat with the remaining pieces.

2 Add the onions to the pan and sauté for 3 minutes or until soft, using a wooden spatula to scrape the browned bits from the bottom of the pan. Add the garlic and sauté for 1 minute, then add the wine and deglaze the pan for 1 more minute, again using the wooden spatula to scrape any browned bits from the bottom of the pan.

3 Add the tomato paste to the pan while stirring rapidly, then add the cinnamon stick, cloves, allspice berries, bay leaf, black pepper, crushed tomatoes, and hot water. Mix well.

4 Add the beef back to the pan. Stir, then cover and reduce the heat to low. Simmer for 1 hour 30 minutes or until the beef is cooked through and tender, and the sauce has thickened. (If the sauce becomes too dry, add more hot water as needed.)

5 About 10 minutes before the cooking time is complete, add the sea salt and stir. When ready to serve, remove the cinnamon stick, bay leaf, allspice berries, and cloves. Store in the refrigerator for up to 3 days.

TIP
This dish is traditionally served with pasta or rice, but it also pairs well with vegetables such green beans or peas.

EACH SERVING HAS:

Calories **565** • Total fat **44g** • Saturated fat **15g** • Carbohydrate **10g** • Fiber **2g** • Protein **33g**

Tender, juicy pork is cooked in wine along with carrots, peppers, and tomatoes to create a delicious and balanced meal. Serve as is, or accompany with rice, couscous, or bread.

ONE-PAN GREEK PORK AND VEGETABLES

 3 SERVINGS   **10 MINUTES**   **40 MINUTES**   **5 OUNCES (140G) PORK WITH ⅔ CUP VEGETABLES**

1lb (450g) pork shoulder, cut into 1-inch (2.5cm) cubes

¾ tsp fine sea salt, divided

½ tsp freshly ground black pepper, divided, plus more for serving

4 tbsp extra virgin olive oil, divided

1 medium red onion, sliced

1 medium green bell pepper, seeded and sliced

1 medium carrot, peeled and julienned

¼ cup dry red wine

15 cherry tomatoes, halved

2 tbsp hot water

½ tsp dried oregano

1   Scatter the cubed pork onto a cutting board and sprinkle with ¼ teaspoon of sea salt and ¼ teaspoon of black pepper. Flip the pieces over and sprinkle an additional ¼ teaspoon of sea salt and the remaining ¼ teaspoon of black pepper.

2   In a large pan wide enough to hold all the pork in a single layer, heat 3 tablespoons of olive oil over high heat. Once the oil is hot, add the pork pieces and brown for 2 minutes, then flip the pork pieces and brown for 2 more minutes. (Do not stir.)

3   Add the onions and sauté for 2 minutes and then add the bell peppers and carrots and sauté for 2 more minutes, ensuring all vegetables are coated with the oil. Reduce the heat to medium, cover the pan loosely, and cook for 5 minutes, stirring occasionally.

4   Add the wine and continue cooking for about 4 minutes, using a wooden spatula to scrape any browned bits from the bottom of the pan. Add about 20 cherry tomato halves and stir gently, then drizzle with the remaining 1 tablespoon of olive oil and add the hot water. Reduce the heat to low and simmer for 15–20 minutes or until all the liquids are absorbed. Remove the pan from the heat.

5   Sprinkle the oregano over the top. Top with the remaining cherry tomato halves and season to taste with the remaining ¼ teaspoon of sea salt and additional black pepper before serving. Store covered in the refrigerator for up to 3 days.

 TIP

If you prefer not to use wine, you can substitute an equal amount of vegetable broth.

EACH SERVING HAS:

Calories **440**   •   Total fat **32g**   •   Saturated fat **10g**   •   Carbohydrate **10g**   •   Fiber **3g**   •   Protein **28g**

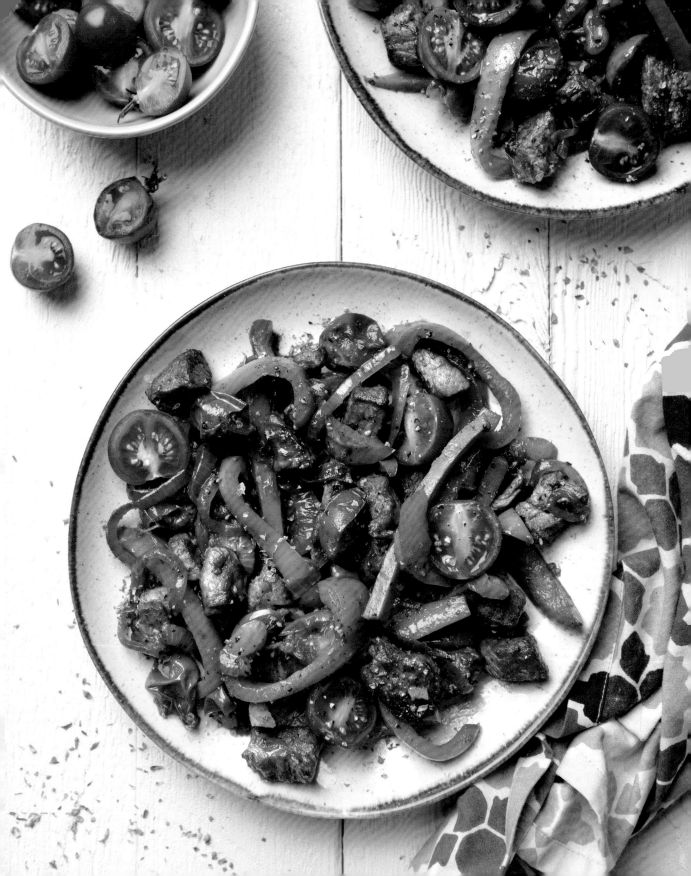

These bite-sized, spiced meatballs are cooked in a rich tomato sauce and are perfect when served over a bed of rice and accompanied with a tossed green salad.

SPICED OVEN-BAKED MEATBALLS
WITH TOMATO SAUCE

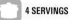 **4 SERVINGS**   **25 MINUTES**   **1 HOUR 5 MINUTES**   **6 MEATBALLS**

1lb (450g) ground chuck

¼ cup unseasoned breadcrumbs

2 garlic cloves, minced

1 tsp salt

½ tsp black pepper

1 tsp ground cumin

3 tbsp chopped fresh parsley

1 egg, lightly beaten

3 tbsp extra virgin olive oil

1 tsp tomato paste

1 tsp red wine vinegar

2 tbsp dry red wine

1 tsp fresh lemon juice

For the sauce

3 medium tomatoes, chopped, or 1 (15oz/425g) can chopped tomatoes

1 tbsp plus 1 tsp tomato paste

¼ cup extra virgin olive oil

1 tsp fine sea salt

¼ tsp black pepper

¼ tsp granulated sugar

1¾ cups hot water

1 Begin making the meatballs by combining all the ingredients in a large bowl. Knead the mixture for 3 minutes or until all the ingredients are well incorporated. Cover the bowl with plastic wrap and transfer the mixture to the refrigerator to rest for at least 20 minutes.

2 While the meatball mixture is resting, preheat the oven to 350°F (175°C) and begin making the sauce by placing all the ingredients except the hot water in a food processor. Process until smooth and then transfer the mixture to a small pan over medium heat. Add the hot water and mix well. Let the mixture come to a boil and then reduce the heat to low and simmer for 10 minutes.

3 Remove the meatball mixture from the refrigerator and shape it into 24 oblong meatballs.

4 Spread 3 tablespoons of the sauce into the bottom of a large baking dish and place the meatballs in a single layer on top of the sauce. Pour the remaining sauce over the top of the meatballs.

5 Bake for 45 minutes or until the meatballs are lightly brown and then turn the meatballs and bake for an additional 10 minutes. (If the sauce appears to be drying out, add another ¼ cup hot water to the baking dish.)

6 Transfer the meatballs to a serving platter. Spoon the sauce over the meatballs before serving. Store covered in the refrigerator for up to 3 days or in an airtight container in the freezer for up to 3 months.

 TIP

To make ahead, prepare the sauce and meat early in the day, and store in the refrigerator until ready to cook.

EACH SERVING HAS:

Calories **560** • Total fat **47g** • Saturated fat **13g** • Carbohydrate **12g** • Fiber **2g** • Protein **22g**

These traditional Greek beef patties are seasoned with herbs and onions, and topped with feta, tomatoes, and olives. The result is a delicious burger that doesn't need condiments!

BIFTEK!
(MEDITERRANEAN BURGERS)

 4 SERVINGS   **1 HOUR 15 MINUTES**   **8 MINUTES**   **1 PATTY WITH TOPPINGS**

1lb (450g) ground chuck

1 egg, lightly beaten

1 small onion (any variety), quartered

4 tbsp breadcrumbs

1 tsp dried mint

1 tsp dried oregano

2 tbsp chopped fresh parsley

1 tbsp extra virgin olive oil

½ tsp salt

¼ tsp freshly ground black pepper

For the toppings

1 tsp fresh lemon juice

4oz (115g) feta, roughly sliced

8 large fresh basil leaves

1 large tomato, sliced

4 Kalamata olives, pitted and thinly sliced

4 tsp extra virgin olive oil

Pinch of dried oregano

1 Place the ground chuck in a medium bowl and add the egg. Use a fork to mix until the egg is partially absorbed.

2 In a food processor, combine the onion, breadcrumbs, mint, oregano, parsley, olive oil, salt, and black pepper. Pulse until all the ingredients are combined and somewhat smooth.

3 Add the onion mixture to the beef mixture and use your hands to knead the mixture for at least 3 minutes, ensuring all the ingredients are well incorporated. Cover the bowl with plastic wrap and transfer to the refrigerator to rest for 1 hour.

4 Remove the beef from the refrigerator and set aside to rest at room temperature for 10 minutes. Shape the mixture into 4 patties and flatten them until they are ¾ inch (2cm) thick.

5 Place a large grill pan over medium heat. When the pan is hot, place the patties in the pan and cook for about 3–4 minutes per side or until the patties are nicely browned and cooked through.

6 To serve, sprinkle a few drops of lemon juice over each patty, then top each patty with 1 ounce of feta, 2 basil leaves, 1 slice of tomato, and 1 sliced Kalamata olive. Drizzle 1 teaspoon of olive oil over each patty and then sprinkle a pinch of oregano over the patties. Store covered in the refrigerator for up to 3 days.

EACH SERVING HAS:

Calories **477** • Total fat **37g** • Saturated fat **15g** • Carbohydrate **11g** • Fiber **2g** • Protein **26g**

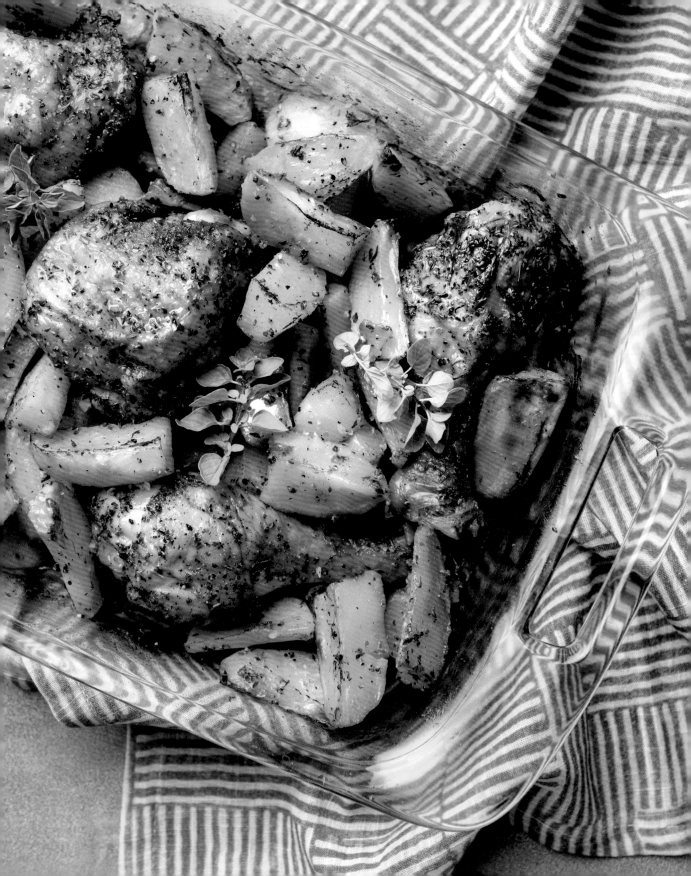

This crispy, flavorful chicken is juicy, oven-roasted with Mediterranean herbs and spices, and accompanied by lemony potatoes.

GREEK ROASTED LEMON CHICKEN
WITH POTATOES

 4 SERVINGS   **10 MINUTES**   **1 HOUR 20 MINUTES**   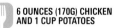 **6 OUNCES (170G) CHICKEN AND 1 CUP POTATOES**

2lb (900g) potatoes (russet or white varieties), peeled

1½lb (680g) chicken pieces (breasts, thighs, legs)

1 cup wine (any variety), for rinsing

1½ tsp freshly ground black pepper, divided

2 tbsp dried oregano, divided

1 tsp salt, divided

½ cup extra virgin olive oil

2 tbsp fresh lemon juice

2 to 3 allspice berries

2 to 3 cloves

2 garlic cloves, cut into quarters

1 Preheat the oven to 375°F (190°C). Place the peeled potatoes in a large bowl and cover them with cold water. Set aside.

2 Rinse the chicken pieces with the wine, pat dry with paper towels, and transfer to a large plate. In a small bowl, mix 1 teaspoon of black pepper, 1 tablespoon of oregano, and ½ teaspoon of salt to make a rub. Apply the rub to the chicken pieces and then set aside.

3 Remove the potatoes from the water. Rinse and pat dry the potatoes, then cut them into wedges and then cut again into half wedges. Place them in a large bowl.

4 Add the olive oil, lemon juice, remaining tablespoon of the oregano, remaining ½ teaspoon of the black pepper, and remaining ½ teaspoon of salt to the potatoes. Mix until all the potatoes are coated with the spices and olive oil.

5 Transfer the potatoes to a large baking dish and spread them into a single layer. Place the chicken pieces on top of the potatoes and then scatter the allspice berries, cloves, and garlic around the chicken.

6 Add hot water to one corner of the dish and then tilt the dish until the water is distributed throughout and fills about ¼ of the depth of the dish. (Do not pour the water directly over the potatoes because it will rinse off the olive oil and spices.)

7 Transfer to the oven and roast for 20 minutes, then reduce the oven temperature to 350°F (180°C) and roast for 1 more hour or until the potatoes and chicken are done. (If the water in the dish evaporates too quickly, add more hot water, ¼ cup at a time.) The potatoes are done when they have a golden color and a knife can be inserted easily. Serve hot. Store in the refrigerator for up to 3 days.

EACH SERVING HAS:

Calories **696** • Total fat **48g** • Saturated fat **9g** • Carbohydrate **31g** • Fiber **4g** • Protein **36g**

Inspired by a popular tapas dish, this moist and flavorful chicken is sautéed with lemon and garlic. It pairs perfectly with a leafy green salad.

SPANISH SAUTÉED LEMON AND GARLIC CHICKEN

 3 SERVINGS   **10 MINUTES**   **15 MINUTES**   **8 OUNCES (30G)**

2 large boneless, skinless chicken breasts (about 1lb/450g)

¼ cup extra virgin olive oil

3 garlic cloves, finely chopped

5 tbsp fresh lemon juice

Zest of 1 lemon

½ cup chopped fresh parsley

¼ tsp fine sea salt

Pinch of freshly ground black pepper

1 Slice the chicken crosswise into very thin slices, each about ¼-inch thick.

2 In a pan large enough to hold the chicken in a single layer, heat the olive oil over medium heat. When the olive oil starts to shimmer, add the garlic and sauté for about 30 seconds, then add the chicken. Reduce the heat to medium-low and sauté for about 12 minutes, tossing the chicken breasts periodically until they begin to brown on the edges.

3 Add the lemon zest and lemon juice. Increase the heat to medium and bring to a boil. Cook for about 2 minutes while using a wooden spatula to scrape any browned bits from the bottom of the pan.

4 Add the parsley, stir, then remove the pan from the heat.

5 Transfer the chicken along with any juices to a platter. Season with the sea salt and black pepper, then serve promptly. Store in an airtight container in the refrigerator for up to 2 days.

 TIP

This chicken is also great when used in salads or on sandwiches.

EACH SERVING HAS:

Calories **316** • Total fat **20g** • Saturated fat **3g** • Carbohydrate **2g** • Fiber **1g** • Protein **31g**

This authentic recipe for the traditional hearty Italian dish features chicken cooked until tender in a zesty sauce of carrots, celery, onions, and tomatoes. Accompany this dish with a green tossed salad or the Cabbage and Carrot Salad (p. 137).

TRADITIONAL CHICKEN CACCIATORE

 4 SERVINGS   **10 MINUTES**   **1 HOUR**   **1 LEG OR THIGH WITH 3 TBSP SAUCE**

1 medium yellow onion, quartered

1 medium carrot, peeled and sliced

1 celery stalk, sliced

2 tbsp extra virgin olive oil

2lb (905g) chicken thighs and legs

½ cup dry red wine

14oz (400g) canned crushed tomatoes

½ tsp fine sea salt

½ cup hot water

Pinch of freshly ground black pepper

1 Combine the onion, carrots, and celery in a food processor. Process until the mixture forms a grainy texture.

2 Add the olive oil to a deep pan over medium heat. When the oil begins to shimmer, add the chicken and sauté until the skin is browned, about 2 minutes per side, then transfer to a plate and set aside.

3 Add the onion and carrot mixture to the pan and sauté for 2–3 minutes, using a wooden spatula to scrape the browned bits from the bottom of the pan. Add the wine to the pan, and continue scraping and deglazing for another 2–3 minutes.

4 Add the crushed tomatoes and sea salt. Mix well, then add the chicken back to the pan along with the hot water. Stir and spoon the sauce over the chicken.

5 Cover, reduce the heat to medium-low, and simmer for about 45 minutes or until the chicken is cooked through and tender, and the sauce has thickened. (Add more hot water in small amounts, as needed, if the sauce begins to dry out.)

6 Transfer the chicken to a plate, spoon the sauce over the chicken, and sprinkle a pinch of black pepper over the top. Allow to cool completely before covering and storing in the refrigerator for up to 2 days.

 TIP
The leftover sauce is wonderful the next day when served over pasta.

EACH SERVING HAS:

Calories **531** • Total fat **34g** • Saturated fat **9g** • Carbohydrate **12g** • Fiber **4g** • Protein **44g**

CHAPTER SIX
SALADS

This perfect Mediterranean salad features simple ingredients but plenty of flavor. This can be enjoyed any time of the day, but it pairs particularly well with fish.

TOSSED GREEN MEDITERRANEAN SALAD

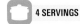 **4 SERVINGS** **15 MINUTES** **NONE** **2 CUPS**

1 medium head romaine lettuce, washed, dried, and chopped into bite-sized pieces

2 medium cucumbers, peeled and sliced

3 spring onions (white parts only), sliced

½ cup finely chopped fresh dill

⅓ cup extra virgin olive oil

2 tbsp fresh lemon juice

¼ tsp fine sea salt

4oz (115g) crumbled feta

7 Kalamata olives, pitted

1 Add the lettuce, cucumber, spring onions, and dill to a large bowl. Toss to combine.

2 In a small bowl, whisk together the olive oil and lemon juice. Pour the dressing over the salad, toss, then sprinkle the sea salt over the top.

3 Sprinkle the feta and olives over the top and then gently toss the salad one more time. Serve promptly. (This recipe is best served fresh.)

TIP

For quicker assembly, wash the lettuce a few hours before serving and store it in the refrigerator.

EACH SERVING HAS:

Calories **323** • Total fat **26g** • Saturated fat **7g** • Carbohydrate **13g** • Fiber **5g** • Protein **8g**

The flavors of the Mediterranean all in one bowl! This refreshing herb salad is made with plenty of fresh parsley and mint mixed with hearty bulgur and then dressed with a tangy lemon vinaigrette.

CLASSIC TABBOULEH

 4 SERVINGS   15 MINUTES   NONE   1¼ CUP

½ cup uncooked bulgur

¾ tsp fine sea salt, divided

1 cup boiling water

2 medium tomatoes (any variety), diced

1 large Persian (or mini) cucumber, diced

2 cups finely chopped fresh parsley

½ cup finely chopped fresh mint

2 spring onions, thinly sliced

½ tsp dried mint leaves

¼ tsp freshly ground black pepper

3 tbsp extra virgin olive oil

3 tbsp fresh lemon juice

1 Combine the bulgur, ¼ teaspoon of the sea salt, and the boiling water in a medium heat-safe bowl. Set aside for 15 minutes.

2 While the bulgur is soaking, combine the tomatoes, cucumbers, parsley, fresh mint, and spring onions in a large bowl. Mix well.

3 In a small bowl, combine the dried mint, remaining ½ teaspoon of the sea salt, black pepper, olive oil, and lemon juice. Stir.

4 Drain the bulgur and then add it to the bowl with the cucumbers and tomatoes. Mix well, then add the dressing and use your hands to mix the ingredients until they're thoroughly combined.

5 Cover the bowl and set it aside for 30 minutes. Serve as a side dish or as a main course. Store covered in the refrigerator for up to 2 days.

EACH SERVING HAS:

Calories **193** • Total fat **11g** • Saturated fat **2g** • Carbohydrate **20g** • Fiber **6g** • Protein **4g**

It's no wonder this is the most popular salad in Greece! Juicy red tomatoes, crisp cucumber, sharp onion, and tangy feta are drizzled with extra virgin olive oil in this flavorful and hearty salad.

TRADITIONAL GREEK SALAD

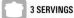 **3 SERVINGS** **10 MINUTES** **NONE** **2 CUPS**

6 tbsp extra virgin olive oil plus 1 tsp for drizzling

3 tbsp red wine vinegar

3 ripe medium tomatoes (any variety), cut into wedges (about 3 cups)

1 medium English cucumber, peeled and sliced

½ small red onion, thinly sliced

½ small green bell pepper, seeded and sliced

¼ tsp fine sea salt

6 Kalamata olives

3oz (85g) slice feta

1 tsp dried oregano

1 In a small bowl, combine the olive oil and vinegar. Whisk and then set aside.

2 Place the tomatoes, cucumbers, onions, and bell peppers in a shallow bowl.

3 Pour the olive oil and vinegar mixture over the salad, then sprinkle the sea salt over the top. Toss gently.

4 Scatter the olives over the salad, then place the slice of feta on top and sprinkle the salad with the oregano.

5 Drizzle 1 teaspoon of the olive oil over the feta before serving. (This salad is best served fresh.)

 TIP
This salad is great as a main course, accompanied with some bread, or served as a side.

EACH SERVING HAS:

Calories **396** • Total fat **37g** • Saturated fat **8g** • Carbohydrate **11g** • Fiber **3g** • Protein **6g**

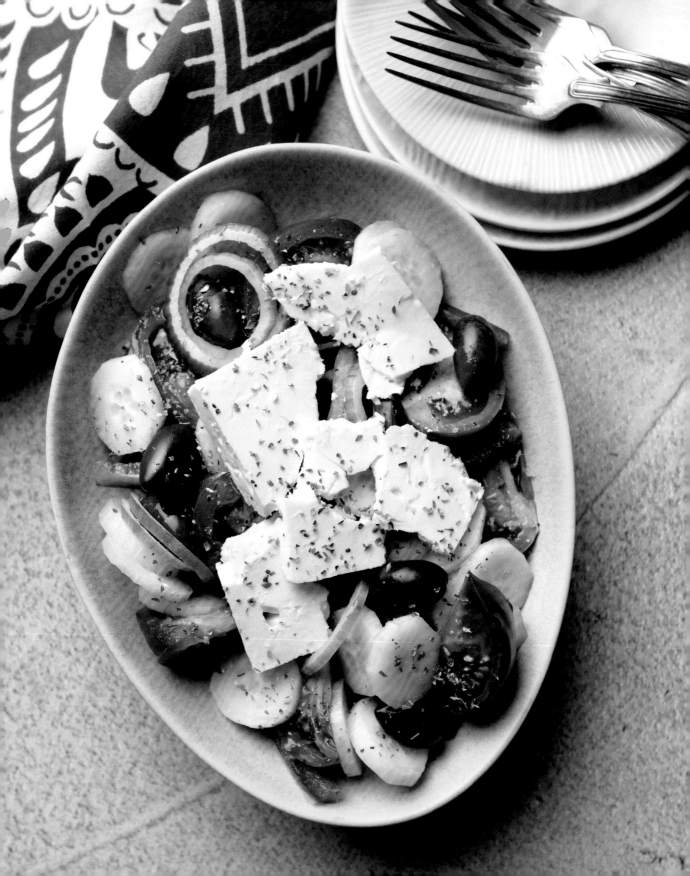

Fresh mozzarella and ripe, firm tomatoes mingle with basil and olive oil in this famous Italian salad, which can be served as a main dish or as an accompaniment.

INSALATA CAPRESE
(ITALIAN TOMATO AND MOZZARELLA SALAD)

 2 SERVINGS   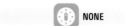 **5 MINUTES**   **NONE**   **½ SALAD**

2 firm medium tomatoes (any variety), cut into ¼-inch (.5cm) slices

¼ tsp kosher salt

8 fresh basil leaves

7oz (200g) fresh mozzarella, cut into ¼-inch (.5cm) slices

¼ tsp dried oregano

3 tsp extra virgin olive oil

1 Place the sliced tomatoes on a cutting board and sprinkle them with the kosher salt. Set aside.

2 Arrange 4 basil leaves in a circular pattern on a large, round serving plate. (Tear the leaves into 2 pieces if they're large.)

3 Assemble the tomato slices and mozzarella slices on top of the basil leaves, alternating a tomato slice and then a mozzarella slice, adding a basil leaf between every 3–4 slices of tomato and mozzarella.

4 Sprinkle the oregano over the top and then drizzle the olive oil over the entire salad. Serve promptly. (This salad is best served fresh.)

 TIP

To avoid a watery salad, make sure the tomatoes are firm and the salad is served promptly, as both the tomatoes and mozzarella often release water after being sliced.

EACH SERVING HAS:

Calories **315** • Total fat **25g** • Saturated fat **13g** • Carbohydrate **5g** • Fiber **2g** • Protein **19g**

Tomatoes, onions, cucumbers, basil, and day-old bread come together to make this flavorful salad. This rustic dish is made with simple ingredients, but it has big flavor.

PANZANELLA
(TUSCAN TOMATO AND BREAD SALAD)

 2 SERVINGS   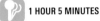 **1 HOUR 5 MINUTES**   **NONE**   **1½ CUPS**

3 tbsp white wine vinegar, divided

1 small red onion, thinly sliced

4oz (115g) stale, dense bread, such as French baguette or Italian (Vienna-style)

1 large tomato (any variety), chopped into bite-sized pieces

1 large Persian (or mini) cucumber, sliced

¼ cup chopped fresh basil

2 tbsp extra virgin olive oil, divided

Pinch of kosher salt

⅛ tsp freshly ground black pepper

1 Add 2 tablespoons of the vinegar to a small bowl filled with water. Add the onion and then set aside.

2 In a medium bowl, combine the remaining tablespoon of vinegar and 2 cups of water. Add the bread to the bowl and soak for 2–3 minutes (depending on how hard the bread is) until the bread has softened on the outside but is not falling apart. Place the bread in a colander and gently squeeze out any excess water and then chop into bite-sized pieces. Arrange the bread pieces on a large plate.

3 Drain the onion and add it to plate with the bread. Add the tomato, cucumber, basil, 1 tablespoon of the olive oil, kosher salt, and black pepper. Toss the ingredients carefully, then cover and transfer to the refrigerator to chill for a minimum of 1 hour.

4 When ready to serve, drizzle the remaining 1 tablespoon of olive oil over the top of the salad and serve promptly. This salad can be stored in the refrigerator for up to 5 hours, but should be consumed on the same day it is prepared.

 TIP

The denser and older the bread, the better. Using a bread that is not dense enough or is too fresh will result in the bread falling apart during the soaking process.

EACH SERVING HAS:

Calories **341** • Total fat **15g** • Saturated fat **2g** • Carbohydrate **43g** • Fiber **4g** • Protein **9g**

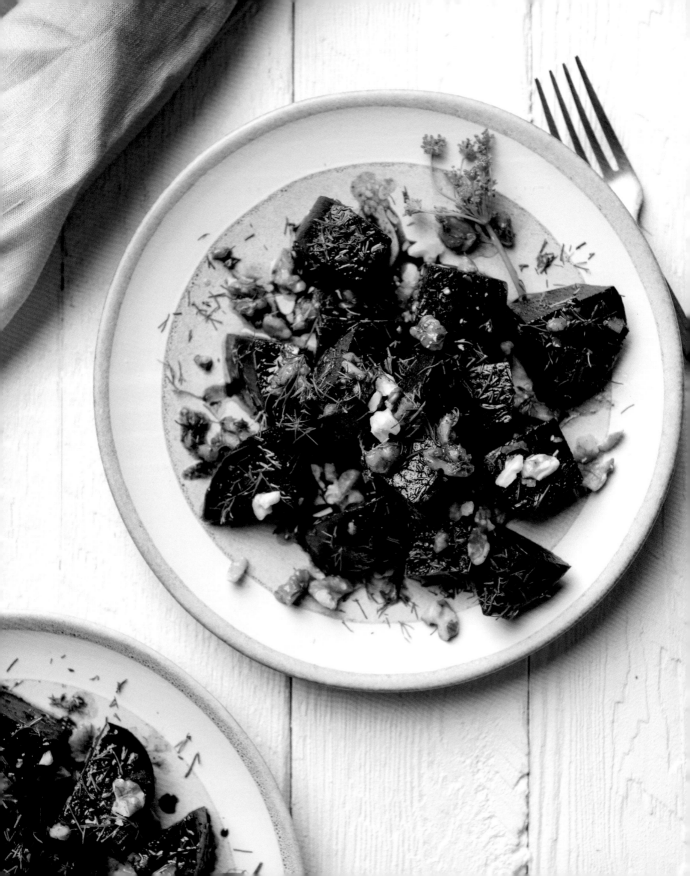

Made with roasted beets, walnuts, and garlic, this delicious and hearty salad is seasoned with fresh dill and an olive oil vinaigrette. It's perfect enjoyed as a side or on its own as a flavorful and nutritious meal.

BEET AND WALNUT SALAD

 2 SERVINGS   5 MINUTES   30 MINUTES   2 CUPS

1lb (450g) fresh beets, trimmed, scrubbed, and peeled

5 tbsp red wine vinegar, divided

4 tbsp extra virgin olive oil

3 garlic cloves, minced

½ cup chopped fresh dill, divided

¼ tsp salt, divided

½ cup chopped walnuts, divided

¼ tsp freshly ground black pepper

1 Place the beets in a large pot. Add 2 tablespoons of the vinegar and fill the pot with enough water to cover the beets, then place the pot over medium heat. Bring to a boil, then cook for 20 to 30 minutes or until the beets are fork-tender. Drain and then set aside to cool.

2 In a small bowl, combine the olive oil and remaining vinegar. Whisk with a fork until the mixture thickens, then add the garlic, ¼ cup of the dill, and ⅛ teaspoon of the salt. Stir to combine.

3 Transfer the cooled beats to a cutting board and cut into 1-inch (2.5cm) cubes.

4 In a large bowl, combine the beets and half of the walnuts, then add the dressing and toss to coat. Top the salad with the remaining walnuts and dill, then season with the black pepper and remaining ⅛ teaspoon of salt. Store in the refrigerator for up to 2 days.

TIP
Feta is a great cheese to pair with this salad.

EACH SERVING HAS:
Calories **561** • Total fat **47g** • Saturated fat **6g** • Carbohydrate **28g** • Fiber **7g** • Protein **8g**

The garlic dressing adds a burst of flavor to this vibrant and refreshing salad. Serve cold along with some hearty bread for soaking up the dressing.

PIPIRRANA
(SPANISH SUMMER SALAD)

 2 SERVINGS   **15 MINUTES**   **NONE**   **2 CUPS**

1 medium red onion, diced

2 large tomatoes, cut into small cubes

1 large Persian or mini cucumber, cut into small cubes

1 large green bell pepper, seeded and diced

2 garlic cloves, minced

Pinch of ground cumin

½ tsp salt plus a pinch for the garlic paste

3 tbsp extra virgin olive oil plus a few drops for the garlic paste

2 tbsp red wine vinegar

1 | Place the onions in a small bowl filled with water. Set aside to soak.

2 | Place the tomatoes, cucumber, and bell pepper in a medium bowl. Drain the onions and then combine them with the rest of the vegetables. Mix well.

3 | In a mortar or small bowl, combine the garlic, cumin, a pinch of salt, and a few drops of olive oil, then roll or mash the ingredients until a paste is formed.

4 | In another small bowl, combine 3 tablespoons of the olive oil, vinegar, and ½ teaspoon of the salt. Add the garlic paste and mix well.

5 | Add the dressing to the salad and mix well.

6 | Cover and refrigerate for 30 minutes before serving. Store in the refrigerator for up to 2 days.

EACH SERVING HAS:

Calories **280** • Total fat **21g** • Saturated fat **3g** • Carbohydrate **19g** • Fiber **5g** • Protein **4g**

This refreshing and light cabbage salad is tossed with shredded carrot and a touch of garlic, and finished with a citrusy olive oil and lemon dressing. This Mediterranean version of coleslaw is perfect for picnics and barbecues.

CABBAGE AND CARROT SALAD

 3 SERVINGS   10 MINUTES   NONE   2 CUPS

½ medium head cabbage, thinly sliced, rinsed, and drained

3 medium carrots, peeled and shredded

4 tbsp extra virgin olive oil

3 tbsp fresh lemon juice

½ tsp salt

¼ tsp freshly ground black pepper

1 garlic clove, minced

8 Kalamata olives, pitted

1 Place the cabbage and carrots in a large bowl and toss.

2 In a jar or small bowl, combine the olive oil, lemon juice, salt, black pepper, and garlic. Whisk or shake to combine.

3 Pour the dressing over the salad and toss. (Note that it will reduce in volume.)

4 Scatter the olives over the salad just before serving. Store covered in the refrigerator for up to 2 days.

 TIP

If you prefer a crunchier salad, add the dressing right before serving.

EACH SERVING HAS:

Calories **268** • Total fat **21g** • Saturated fat **3g** • Carbohydrate **16g** • Fiber **6g** • Protein **3g**

This traditional Cretan dish can be a meal for one or shared as an appetizer. It includes crunchy rusks soaked in olive oil and topped with tomato, feta, capers, and olives.

DAKOS
(CRETAN SALAD)

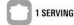 1 SERVING   7 MINUTES   NONE   1 SALAD

1 medium ripe tomato (any variety)

2 whole-grain crispbreads or rusks (or 1 slice toasted whole-grain, wheat, or barley bread)

1 tbsp plus 1 tsp extra virgin olive oil

Pinch of kosher salt

1.5oz (40g) crumbled feta

2 tsp capers, drained

2 Kalamata olives, pitted

Pinch of dried oregano

1 Slice a thin round off the bottom of the tomato. Hold the tomato from the stem side and begin grating the tomato over a plate, using the largest holes of the grater. Grate until only the skin of the tomato remains, then discard the skin. Use a fine mesh strainer to drain the liquid from the grated tomato.

2 Place the crisps on a plate, one next to the other, and sprinkle with a few drops of water. Drizzle 1 tablespoon of the olive oil over the crisps and then top the crisps with the grated tomato, ensuring the crisps are thoroughly covered with the tomato.

3 Sprinkle the kosher salt over the tomato, then layer the crumbled feta over the top. Top with the capers and olives, and sprinkle the oregano over the top and drizzle with the remaining 1 teaspoon of olive oil. Serve promptly. (This salad is best served fresh.)

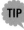 TIP
Traditionally, this salad is made using whole-grain barley rusks, which are made from double-baked bread. They're available to order online or at Greek grocery stores.

EACH SERVING HAS:

Calories **425** • Total fat **29g** • Saturated fat **9g** • Carbohydrate **28g** • Fiber **6g** • Protein **11g**

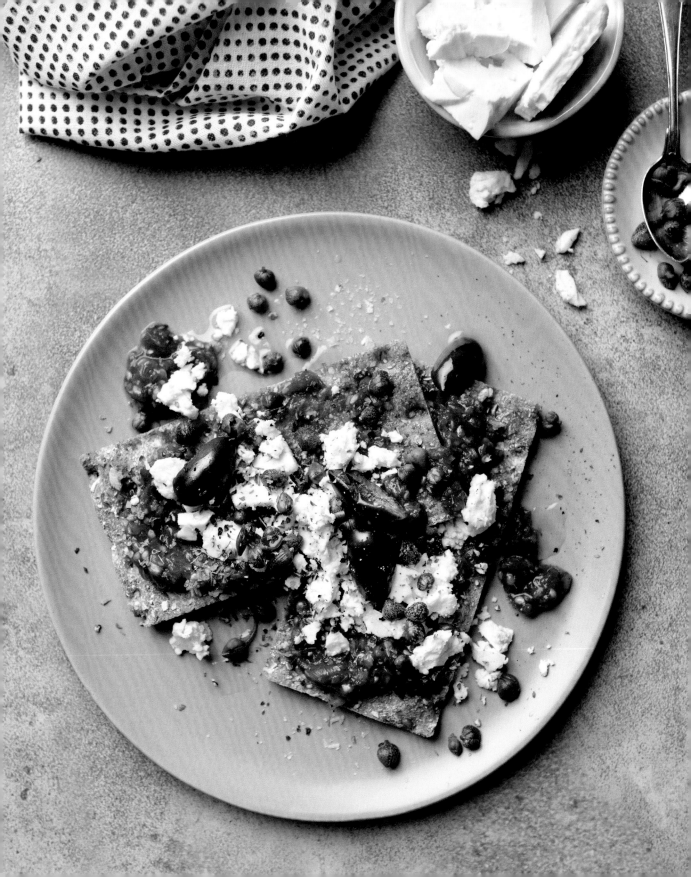

This refreshing and light salad is made with crispy raw zucchini and herbed ricotta, and finished with a tangy lemon vinaigrette and a sprinkle of toasted pine nuts. The delicate flavor of the zucchini stands out, while the pine nuts add extra crunch.

ZUCCHINI AND RICOTTA SALAD

 1 SERVING   **5 MINUTES** 🕐 **2 MINUTES** 🍴 **1¾ CUP**

2 tsp raw pine nuts

5oz (140g) whole-milk ricotta cheese

1 tbsp chopped fresh mint

1 tsp chopped fresh basil

1 tbsp chopped fresh parsley

Pinch of fine sea salt

1 medium zucchini (about 3oz/85g), very thinly sliced horizontally with a mandoline slicer

Pinch of freshly ground black pepper

For the dressing

1½ tbsp extra virgin olive oil

1 tbsp fresh lemon juice

Pinch of fine sea salt

Pinch of freshly ground black pepper

1 Add the pine nuts to a small pan placed over medium heat. Toast the nuts, turning them frequently, for 2 minutes or until golden. Set aside.

2 In a food processor, combine the ricotta, mint, basil, parsley, and a pinch of sea salt. Process until smooth and then set aside.

3 Make the dressing by combining the olive oil and lemon juice in a small bowl. Use a fork to stir rapidly until the mixture thickens, then add a pinch of sea salt and a pinch of black pepper. Stir again.

4 Place the sliced zucchini in a medium bowl. Add half of the dressing, and toss to coat the zucchini.

5 To serve, place half of the ricotta mixture in the center of a serving plate, then layer the zucchini in a circle, covering the cheese. Add the rest of the cheese in the center and on top of the zucchini, then sprinkle the toasted pine nuts over the top. Drizzle the remaining dressing over the top, and finish with a pinch of black pepper. Store covered in the refrigerator for up to 1 day.

EACH SERVING HAS:

Calories **490** • Total fat **43g** • Saturated fat **15g** • Carbohydrate **8g** • Fiber **2g** • Protein **18g**

This salad is a perfect fruit and cheese combination! The crisp watermelon is paired with tangy feta and finished with a simple honey balsamic dressing.

WATERMELON AND FETA SALAD

 2 SERVINGS   5 MINUTES   NONE   1 CUP

2 cups cubed watermelon

2oz (55g) feta, cubed

¼ cup chopped fresh mint

1 tsp extra virgin olive oil

2 tsp balsamic vinegar

½ tsp honey

Pinch of coarse sea salt

2 tsp sesame seeds

¼ tsp freshly ground
   black pepper

1 Place the watermelon, feta, and mint in a medium bowl. Toss gently.

2 Combine the olive oil, vinegar, honey, and sea salt in a small bowl, and mix.

3 Drizzle the dressing over the salad and toss. Sprinkle the sesame seeds and black pepper over the top of the salad.

4 Cover and transfer to the refrigerator to rest for 1 hour before serving. (Do not drain the salad.) This salad is best served fresh on the same day it's prepared and will not keep well in the refrigerator.

 TIP

The watermelon will release juices while the salad is resting in the fridge, but you should not drain them from the salad because that will also drain the dressing.

EACH SERVING HAS:

Calories **187** • Total fat **11g** • Saturated fat **5g** • Carbohydrate **16g** • Fiber **2g** • Protein **6g**

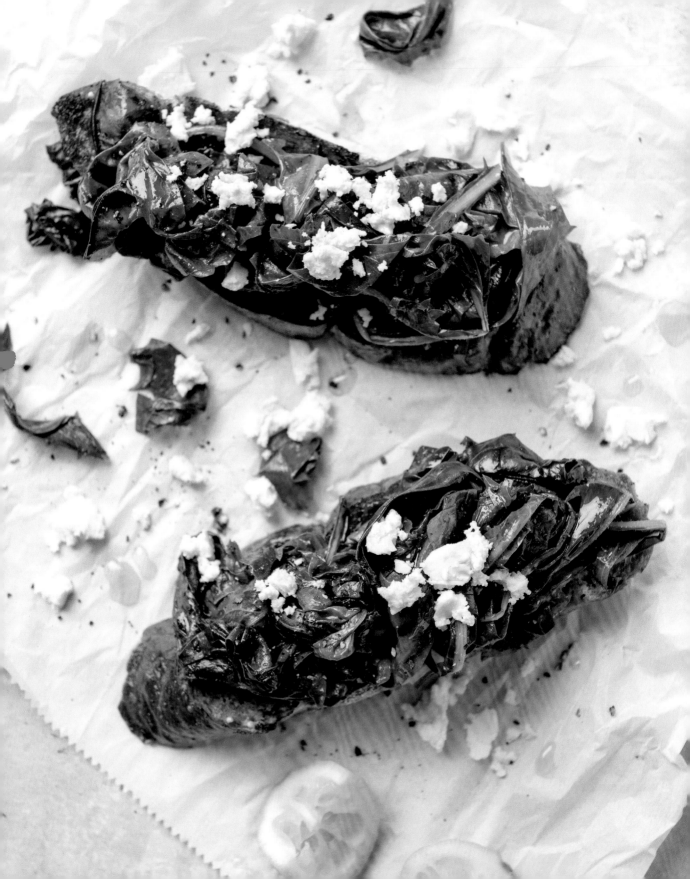

A Mediterranean superfood! The greens are cooked until tender, dressed with olive oil and fresh lemon juice, and served with tangy feta atop hearty bread.

HORTA
(WARM GREENS SALAD)

 2 SERVINGS   **5 MINUTES**   **15 MINUTES**   **1 SLICE OF BREAD AND 1 CUP GREENS**

¼ tsp fine sea salt

1lb (450g) greens (dandelion, mustard, collard, endive, or chard), washed and trimmed

3 tbsp extra virgin olive oil plus 1 tsp for drizzling

2 tbsp fresh lemon juice

2 slices whole-wheat bread

2 tbsp crumbled feta

2 pinches of freshly ground black pepper

Pinch of kosher salt for serving

1 Fill a large pot with water and place over high heat. When the water begins to boil, add the sea salt and greens and then reduce the heat to medium. Continue boiling, uncovered, for 10–15 minutes or until the greens are soft and the stems are tender, then drain and transfer the greens to a large bowl.

2 Make the dressing by combining the olive oil and lemon juice in a small bowl. Whisk with a fork.

3 Add the dressing to the greens and toss until the greens are coated.

4 Toast the bread slices and place them on two serving plates. Top each slice with 1 cup of the greens, 1 tablespoon of the feta, a pinch of the black pepper, and ½ teaspoon of the olive oil. Sprinkle a pinch of kosher salt over the top before serving. Store the greens only in the refrigerator for up to 3 days.

TIP

The cooking water for the greens can be enjoyed as a warm, nutrient-rich beverage.

EACH SERVING HAS:

Calories **493** • Total fat **34g** • Saturated fat **8g** • Carbohydrate **34g** • Fiber **10g** • Protein **13g**

Peppery arugula and baby spinach are paired with Parmesan, sweet dried figs, and a honey balsamic vinaigrette. Toasted pine nuts give this salad crunch.

ARUGULA SPINACH SALAD
WITH SHAVED PARMESAN

 3 SERVINGS   **10 MINUTES**   **2 MINUTES**   **1½ CUPS**

3 tbsp raw pine nuts

3 cups arugula

3 cups baby leaf spinach

5 dried figs, pitted and chopped

2.5oz (70g) shaved Parmesan cheese

For the dressing

4 tsp balsamic vinegar

1 tsp Dijon mustard

1 tsp honey

5 tbsp extra virgin olive oil

1 In a small pan over low heat, toast the pine nuts for 2 minutes or until they begin to brown. Promptly remove them from the heat and transfer to a small bowl.

2 Make the dressing by combining the balsamic vinegar, Dijon mustard, and honey in a small bowl. Using a fork to whisk, gradually add the olive oil while continuously mixing.

3 In a large bowl, toss the arugula and baby spinach and then top with the figs, Parmesan cheese, and toasted pine nuts. Drizzle the dressing over the top and toss until the ingredients are thoroughly coated with the dressing. Serve promptly. (This salad is best served fresh.)

EACH SERVING HAS:

Calories **365** • Total fat **31g** • Saturated fat **7g** • Carbohydrate **14g** • Fiber **3g** • Protein **11g**

Potatoes and onions are gently marinated in olive oil and red wine vinegar and then finished with a sprinkle of oregano in this flavorful salad. Serve as a side or as a meal.

MEDITERRANEAN NO-MAYO POTATO SALAD

 4 SERVINGS   **5 MINUTES**   **15 MINUTES**   **1 CUP**

2lb (905g) potatoes (white or Yukon Gold varieties), peeled and cut into 1½-inch (3.75cm) chunks

¼ cup extra virgin olive oil

3 tbsp red wine vinegar

½ medium red onion, chopped

2 tbsp dried oregano

½ tsp fine sea salt

1 Fill a medium pot with water and place it over high heat. When the water comes to a boil, carefully place the potatoes in the water, reduce the heat to medium, and simmer for 12–15 minutes or until the potatoes can be pierced with a fork but are not falling apart. Use a slotted spoon to transfer the potatoes to a colander, rinse briefly with cold water, then set aside to drain.

2 In a small bowl, whisk the olive oil and red wine vinegar.

3 Transfer the potatoes to a large bowl. Add the olive oil and vinegar mixture to the potatoes and toss gently and then add the onions. Rub the oregano between your fingers to release the aroma, then sprinkle it over the potatoes and toss again. Add the sea salt and toss once more. Store in an airtight container in the refrigerator for up to 3 days.

 TIP

This salad can be served right away; however, the longer the potatoes marinate in the dressing, the more flavorful the salad will become.

EACH SERVING HAS:

Calories **266** • Total fat **14g** • Saturated fat **2g** • Carbohydrate **30g** • Fiber **4g** • Protein **5g**

This simple salad features intense flavors. Fresh tomatoes are paired with capers, green olives, and red onions, and then dressed with extra virgin olive oil. Enjoy it as a first course, or pair it with a bowl of your favorite pasta.

SICILIAN SALAD

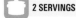 2 SERVINGS   5 MINUTES   NONE   1¼ CUPS

2 tbsp extra virgin olive oil

1 tbsp red wine vinegar

2 medium tomatoes (preferably beefsteak variety), sliced

½ medium red onion, thinly sliced

2 tbsp capers, drained

6 green olives, halved

1 tsp dried oregano

Pinch of fine sea salt

1 | Make the dressing by combining the olive oil and vinegar in a small bowl. Use a fork to whisk until the mixture thickens slightly. Set aside.

2 | Arrange the sliced tomatoes on a large plate and then scatter the onions, capers, and olives over the tomatoes.

3 | Sprinkle the oregano and sea salt over the top, then drizzle the dressing over the salad. Serve promptly. (This salad is best served fresh, but can be stored covered in the refrigerator for up to 1 day.)

EACH SERVING HAS:

Calories **183** • Total fat **16g** • Saturated fat **2g** • Carbohydrate **8g** • Fiber **3g** • Protein **2g**

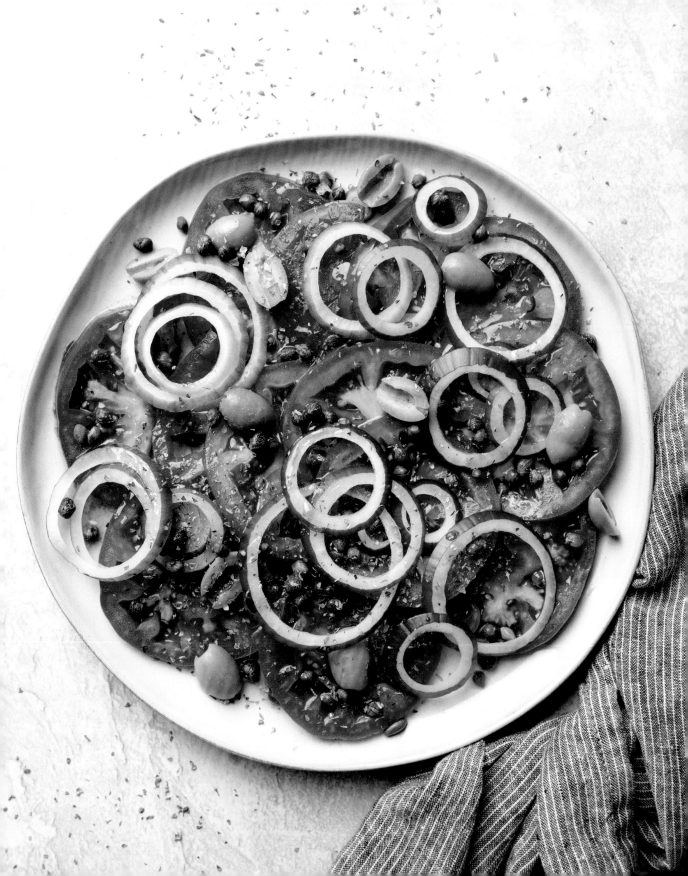

The richness of the avocado pairs well with the citrus in this salad. The olive oil and cumin dressing balances out the flavors while providing a warm and earthy aroma. It's a tangy and refreshing salad that makes a filling and flavorful lunch.

CITRUS AVOCADO SALAD

 2 SERVINGS   5 MINUTES   NONE   1½ CUPS

½ medium orange (any variety), peeled and cut into bite-sized chunks

1 medium tangerine, peeled and sectioned

½ medium white grapefruit, peeled and cut into bite-sized chunks

2 thin slices red onion

1 medium avocado, peeled, pitted, and sliced

Pinch of freshly ground black pepper

For the dressing

3 tbsp extra virgin olive oil

1 tbsp fresh lemon juice

½ tsp ground cumin

½ tsp coarse sea salt

Pinch of freshly ground black pepper

1 Make the dressing by combining the olive oil, lemon juice, cumin, sea salt, and black pepper in a small jar or bowl. Whisk or shake to combine.

2 Toss the orange, tangerine, and grapefruit in a medium bowl, then place the sliced onion on top. Drizzle half the dressing over the salad.

3 Fan the avocado slices over the top of the salad. Drizzle the remaining dressing over the salad and then sprinkle a pinch of black pepper over the top.

4 Toss gently before serving. (This salad is best eaten fresh, but can be stored in the refrigerator for up to 1 day.)

 TIP
For a slightly sweeter salad, substitute red or pink grapefruit for the white grapefruit.

EACH SERVING HAS:

Calories **380** • Total fat **31g** • Saturated fat **4g** • Carbohydrate **24g** • Fiber **7g** • Protein **3g**

Barley, zucchini, tomatoes, herbs, and olives come together in this refreshing and hearty traditional Italian summer salad that is finished with a lemon vinaigrette.

ITALIAN SUMMER VEGETABLE BARLEY SALAD

 4 SERVINGS   **10 MINUTES**    **25–40 MINUTES**   **1½ CUPS**

1 cup uncooked barley (hulled or pearl)

3 cups water

¾ tsp fine sea salt, divided

1 tsp plus 3 tbsp extra virgin olive oil, divided

3 tbsp fresh lemon juice

2 medium zucchini, washed and chopped

15 Kalamata olives, pitted and sliced or chopped

¼ cup chopped fresh parsley

¼ cup chopped fresh basil

1 cup cherry tomatoes, halved

½ tsp freshly ground black pepper

1 Place the barley in a medium pot and add 3 cups of water and ¼ teaspoon of the sea salt. Bring to a boil over high heat, then reduce the heat to low. Simmer for 25–40 minutes, depending on the type of barley you're using, adding small amounts of hot water if the barley appears to be drying out. Cook until the barley is soft but still chewy, then transfer to a mesh strainer and rinse with cold water.

2 Empty the rinsed barley into a large bowl, drizzle 1 teaspoon of the olive oil over the top, fluff with a fork, and then set aside.

3 In a small bowl, combine the remaining 3 tablespoons of olive oil and the lemon juice. Whisk until the dressing thickens.

4 In a large bowl, combine the barley, zucchini, olives, parsley, and basil. Toss and then add the cherry tomatoes, remaining ½ teaspoon of sea salt, and black pepper. Toss gently, drizzle the dressing over the top, and continue tossing until the ingredients are coated with the dressing. Serve promptly. Store covered in the refrigerator for up to 3 days.

TIP
Hulled barley is the whole-grain form of barley and maintains most of its nutrients and fiber, compared to pearl barley.

EACH SERVING HAS:

Calories **328** • Total fat **17g** • Saturated fat **2g** • Carbohydrate **39g** • Fiber **9g** • Protein **7g**

CHAPTER SEVEN

SNACKS AND APPETIZERS

These little fish have big flavor and contain loads of mood-boosting omega-3's! The tangy and savory topping is made with flavorful capers, onions, and sardines, and is layered on crusty whole-wheat bread. This is great as a healthy snack or a hearty hors d'oeuvre.

SARDINE AND HERB BRUSCHETTA

 4 SERVINGS   **5 MINUTES**   🕐 **10 MINUTES**   🍴 **2 SLICES**

8 (1-inch/2.5cm) thick whole-grain baguette slices

1½ tbsp extra virgin olive oil

4oz (115g) olive oil–packed sardines (about 1 can)

2 tbsp fresh lemon juice

1 tsp red wine vinegar

2 tbsp capers, drained

3 tbsp finely chopped onion (any variety)

½ tsp dried oregano

1 tbsp finely chopped fresh mint

1 garlic clove, halved

1 Preheat the oven to 400°F (200°C).

2 Place the baguette slices on a large baking sheet and brush them with the olive oil. Transfer to the oven and toast until the slices are golden, about 10 minutes.

3 While the baguette slices are toasting, make the sardine topping by combining the sardines, lemon juice, and vinegar in a medium bowl. Mash with a fork. Add the capers, onions, oregano, and mint, and stir to combine.

4 When the baguette slices are done toasting, remove them from the oven and rub them with the garlic.

5 Transfer the slices to a serving platter. Place 1 heaping tablespoon of the topping onto each baguette slice. Store the sardine topping in the refrigerator for up to 3 days.

TIP
This topping is also great as a lunch when served on a large slice of toasted whole-grain bread along with a salad.

EACH SERVING HAS:

Calories **193** • Total fat **9g** • Saturated fat **1g** • Carbohydrate **16g** • Fiber **2g** • Protein **11g**

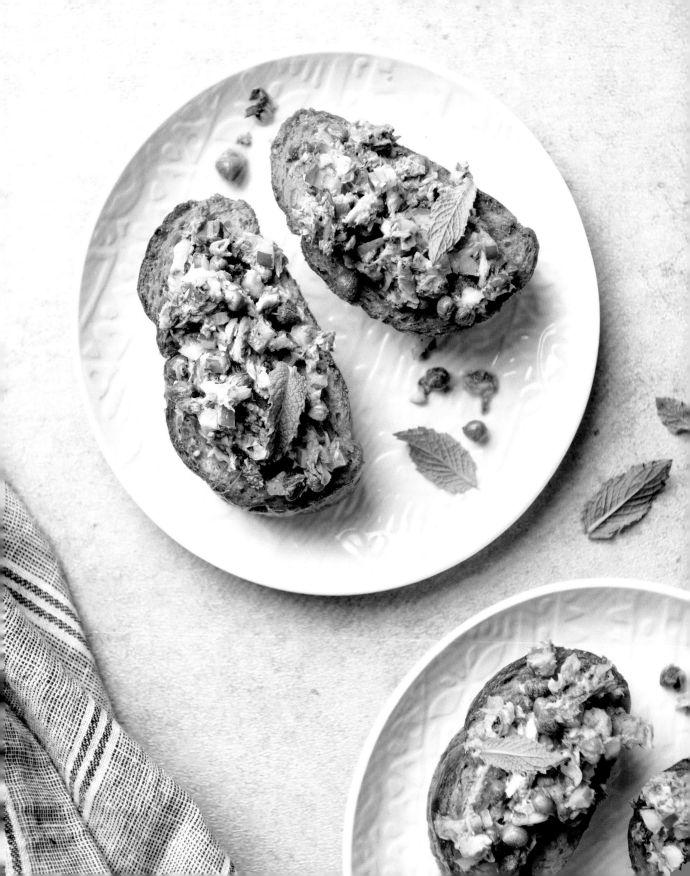

This simple homemade tapenade is made from flavorful Kalamata olives, capers, and garlic. It makes for a great spread, dip, or even a topping for pasta. Or use it as a substitute for mayonnaise on sandwiches for a dose of healthy fats.

KALAMATA OLIVE TAPENADE

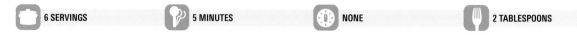

| | 6 SERVINGS | | 5 MINUTES | | NONE | | 2 TABLESPOONS |

7oz (200g) Kalamata olives (about 30), pitted and drained

2 tbsp capers, rinsed and drained

2 tsp dried oregano

2 garlic cloves, minced

1 Combine the ingredients in a food processor and pulse, using a spatula to scrape the sides, until all the ingredients form a chunky paste.

2 Store in an airtight jar in the refrigerator for up to 2 weeks.

EACH SERVING HAS:

Calories **65** • Total fat **7g** • Saturated fat **1g** • Carbohydrate **1g** • Fiber **1g** • Protein **0g**

These mushrooms are filled with a combination of fresh herbs and a bit of tangy feta cheese for a simple, yet tasty, version of this classic appetizer.

MEDiTERRANEAN-STYLE STUFFED MUSHROOMS

 4 SERVINGS   **10 MINUTES**   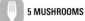 **20 MINUTES**   **5 MUSHROOMS**

2oz (55g) feta

1 tbsp cream cheese

2 tsp dried oregano

1 tbsp finely chopped
   fresh parsley

2 tbsp finely chopped
   fresh basil

2 tbsp finely chopped
   fresh mint

¼ tsp freshly ground
   black pepper

3 tbsp unseasoned
   breadcrumbs, divided

2 tbsp extra virgin olive oil,
   divided

20 medium button
   mushrooms (about
   12oz/340g), washed, dried,
   and stems removed

1 Preheat the oven to 400°F (200°C). Line a large baking pan with foil.

2 In a medium bowl, combine the feta, cream cheese, oregano, parsley, basil, mint, black pepper, 2 tablespoons of the breadcrumbs, and 1 tablespoon of the olive oil. Use a fork to mash the ingredients until they're combined and somewhat creamy.

3 Stuff the mushrooms with the filling and then place them in the prepared pan.

4 Sprinkle the remaining 1 tablespoon of breadcrumbs over the mushrooms and then drizzle the remaining olive oil over the top.

5 Bake for 15–20 minutes or until the tops are golden brown. Serve promptly.

 TIP
You can make the filling ahead of time and store it covered in the refrigerator for up to 2 days.

EACH SERVING HAS:

Calories **143** • Total fat **10g** • Saturated fat **3g** • Carbohydrate **9g** • Fiber **1g** • Protein **5g**

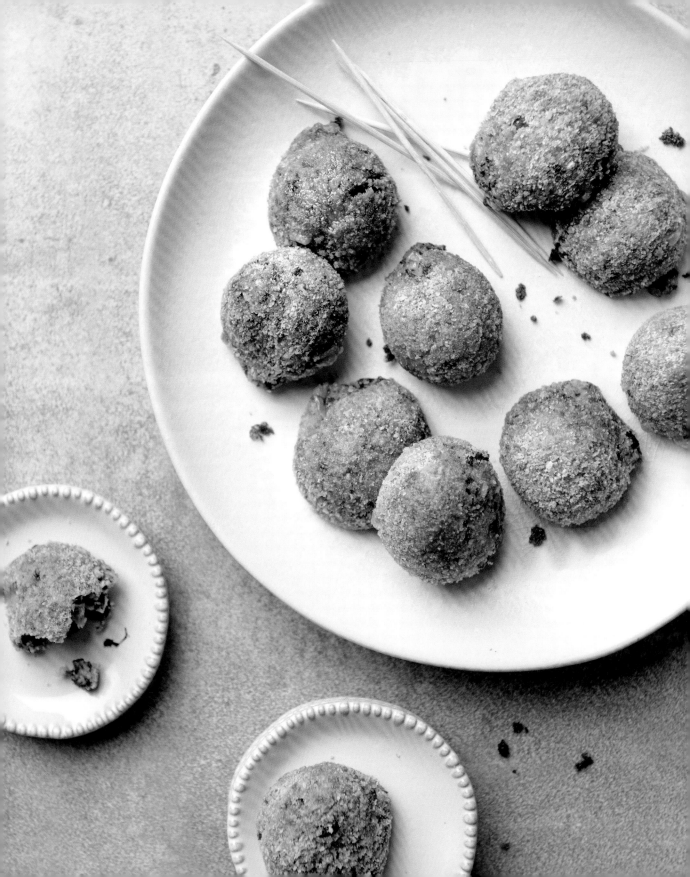

A classic flavor combination comes together in these tasty morsels: melted ricotta and sautéed spinach are coated in a crispy breadcrumb crust and then baked until golden.

BAKED ITALIAN SPINACH AND RICOTTA BALLS

 4 SERVINGS   **15 MINUTES**   **26 MINUTES**   **5 BALLS**

1½ tbsp extra virgin olive oil

1 garlic clove

9oz (255g) fresh baby leaf spinach, washed

3 spring onions (white parts only), thinly sliced

9oz (255g) ricotta, drained

1.75oz (50g) grated Parmesan cheese

2 tbsp chopped fresh basil

¾ tsp salt, divided

¼ tsp plus a pinch of freshly ground black pepper, divided

4½ tbsp plus ⅓ cup unseasoned breadcrumbs, divided

1 egg

1 Preheat the oven to 400°F (200°C). Line a large baking pan with parchment paper.

2 Add the olive oil and garlic clove to a large pan over medium heat. When the oil begins to shimmer, add the spinach and sauté, tossing continuously, until the spinach starts to wilt, then add the spring onions. Continue tossing and sautéing until most of the liquid has evaporated, about 6 minutes, then transfer the spinach and onion mixture to a colander to drain and cool for 10 minutes.

3 When the spinach mixture has cooled, discard the garlic clove and squeeze the spinach to remove as much of the liquid as possible. Transfer the spinach mixture to a cutting board and finely chop.

4 Combine the ricotta, Parmesan, basil, ½ teaspoon of the salt, and ¼ teaspoon of the black pepper in a large bowl. Use a fork to mash the ingredients together, then add the spinach and continue mixing until the ingredients are combined. Add 4½ tablespoons of the breadcrumbs and mix until all ingredients are well combined.

5 In a small bowl, whisk the egg with the remaining ¼ teaspoon salt and a pinch of the black pepper. Place the remaining ⅓ cup of breadcrumbs on a small plate. Scoop out 1 tablespoon of the spinach mixture and roll it into a smooth ball, then dip it in the egg mixture and then roll it in the breadcrumbs. Place the ball on the prepared baking pan and continue the process with the remaining spinach mixture.

6 Bake for 16–20 minutes or until the balls turn a light golden brown. Remove the balls from the oven and serve promptly. Store covered in the refrigerator for up to 1 day. (Reheat before serving.)

EACH SERVING HAS:

Calories **243** • Total fat **13g** • Saturated fat **8g** • Carbohydrate **16g** • Fiber **2g** • Protein **16g**

These delightful Mediterranean-inspired pizzas are topped with a citrusy tahini sauce, tomatoes, artichoke hearts, olives, and more. They're easy to make and delicious!

LOADED VEGETABLE PITA PIZZAS
WITH TAHINI SAUCE

 2 SERVINGS   **5 MINUTES**   🕐 **12 MINUTES**   🍴 **1 PIZZA**

2 (6-inch/15.25cm) pita breads

4 canned artichoke hearts, chopped

¼ cup chopped tomato (any variety)

¼ cup chopped onion (any variety)

4 Kalamata olives, pitted and sliced

4 green olives, pitted and sliced

2 tsp pine nuts

2 tsp extra virgin olive oil

Pinch of kosher salt

Juice of 1 lemon

For the tahini sauce

2 tbsp tahini

2 tbsp fresh lemon juice

1 tbsp water

1 garlic clove, minced

Pinch of freshly ground black pepper

1 Preheat the oven to 400°F (200°C) and line a large baking sheet with wax paper.

2 Make the tahini sauce by combining the tahini and lemon juice in a small bowl. While stirring rapidly, begin adding the water, garlic, and black pepper. Continue stirring rapidly until the ingredients are well combined and smooth.

3 Place the pita breads on the prepared baking sheet. Spread about 1 tablespoon of the tahini sauce over the top of each pita and then top each pita with the chopped artichoke hearts, 2 tablespoons of the tomatoes, 2 tablespoons of the onions, half of the sliced Kalamata olives, half of the green olives, and 1 teaspoon of the pine nuts.

4 Transfer the pizzas to the oven and bake for 12 minutes or until the edges of the pita breads turn golden and crunchy.

5 Drizzle 1 teaspoon of the olive oil over each pizza, then sprinkle a pinch of kosher salt over the top followed by a squeeze of lemon. Cut the pizzas into quarters. Store covered in the refrigerator for up to 2 days.

 TIP
If desired, top the each pizza with 2 to 3 teaspoons of crumbled feta.

EACH SERVING HAS:

Calories **423** • Total fat **23g** • Saturated fat **3g** • Carbohydrate **44g** • Fiber **5g** • Protein **10g**

Lentils get a boost of flavor with the addition of Kalamata olives, capers, and tuna. Serve this hearty bowl as a meal or as an appetizer along with some whole-grain crackers. It's also a great way to use up leftover lentil stew.

MEDITERRANEAN LENTIL BOWL

 2 SERVINGS   **5 MINUTES**   **45 MINUTES**   **1 CUP**

½ cup uncooked brown lentils

½ medium onion (any variety), chopped

1 garlic clove, halved

1 bay leaf

1 tsp tomato paste

1¼ cups hot water

3 cherry tomatoes, sliced

2 Kalamata olives, rinsed, pitted, and sliced

2 tsp capers, rinsed and drained

¼ cup water-packed canned tuna

2 oil-packed sun-dried tomatoes, rinsed and roughly chopped

2 tsp extra virgin olive oil

1 tsp balsamic vinegar

½ tsp dried oregano

1 In a medium pot, combine the lentils, onions, garlic, bay leaf, tomato paste, and the hot water. Bring to a boil and then reduce the heat to low and simmer for 25 minutes, checking the water levels intermittently to ensure the lentils aren't too dry. (If the lentils aren't done after 25 minutes, add ¼ cup hot water and continue simmering for 15–20 minutes or until the lentils are soft.) Remove from the heat, and discard the bay leaf and garlic clove. Set aside to cool for 10 minutes.

2 In a medium bowl, combine the cooked lentils, tomatoes, olives, capers, tuna, sun-dried tomatoes, olive oil, and balsamic vinegar. Stir to combine.

3 Sprinkle the oregano over the top before serving. Store in the refrigerator for up to 2 days.

EACH SERVING HAS:

Calories **276** • Total fat **7g** • Saturated fat **1g** • Carbohydrate **33g** • Fiber **16g** • Protein **20g**

These roasted, caramelized dates are stuffed with feta and Parmesan. They're a satisfying treat that combines both sweet and salty flavors.

STUFFED DATES
WITH FETA, PARMESAN, AND PINE NUTS

 4 SERVINGS   **5 MINUTES**   **10 MINUTES**   🍴 **3 DATES**

1oz (30g) feta

1oz (30g) Parmesan cheese

12 dried dates, pitted

½ tbsp raw pine nuts

1 tsp extra virgin olive oil

1 | Preheat the oven to 425°F (220°C). Line a small baking pan with parchment paper.

2 | Cut the feta and Parmesan into 12 small thin sticks, each about ¾ inch (2cm) long and ¼ inch (.5cm) thick.

3 | Use a sharp knife to cut a small slit lengthwise into each date. Insert a piece of the Parmesan followed by a piece of the feta, and then press 2–3 pine nuts slightly into the feta.

4 | Transfer the dates to the prepared baking pan and place in the oven to roast for 10 minutes. (The edges of the dates should begin to brown.)

5 | Remove the dates from the oven and drizzle a few drops of the olive oil over each date. Serve promptly. (These do not store well and are best enjoyed fresh.)

EACH SERVING HAS:

Calories **127** • Total fat **5g** • Saturated fat **2g** • Carbohydrate **16g** • Fiber **2g** • Protein **4g**

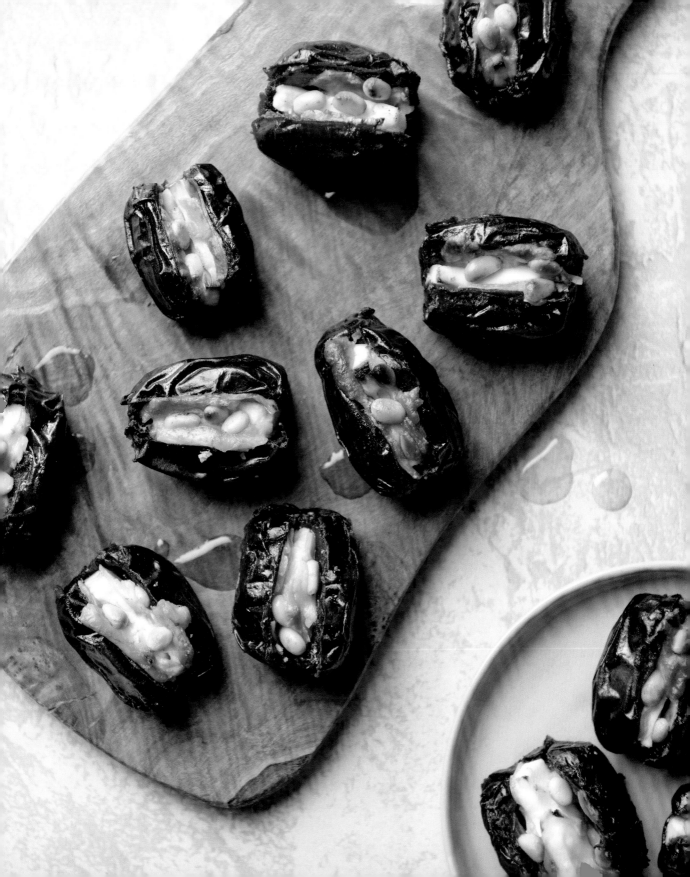

This delicious spread is made with chickpeas, tahini, and lemon. It's rich in protein and fiber, and perfect for dipping bread or vegetables, or for spreading on a sandwich in place of mayonnaise.

CLASSIC HUMMUS

 8 SERVINGS   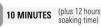 **10 MINUTES** (plus 12 hours soaking time)   **20–40 MINUTES**   **3 TABLESPOONS**

¾ cup uncooked chickpeas

½ tsp baking soda

¼ cup tahini

3⅓ tbsp fresh lemon juice, divided

4–5 tbsp reserved chickpea cooking water, divided

1 garlic clove, crushed

¼ tsp fine sea salt

1 tsp extra virgin olive oil

1 Place the chickpeas in a large bowl and cover with water by 3 inches to allow for expansion. Add the baking soda. Set aside to soak for 12 hours or overnight.

2 When ready to cook, drain and rinse the chickpeas and transfer to a large pot. Cover with cold water and bring to a boil over medium-high heat, removing any foam with a slotted spoon, then reduce the heat to low and simmer until soft and tender, about 20–40 minutes. Reserve ½ cup of the cooking water and then drain the chickpeas.

3 Combine the tahini, 3 tablespoons of the lemon juice, and 2 tablespoons of the cooking water in a food processor. Process until smooth.

4 Add the chickpeas, garlic, and sea salt to a food processor. Process until smooth, gradually adding the remaining 2–3 tablespoons of cooking water until the mixture becomes light and creamy. Taste and add additional salt and lemon juice as needed.

5 Transfer the hummus to a bowl, and drizzle the olive oil over the top before serving. Store covered in the refrigerator for up to 4 days.

EACH SERVING HAS:

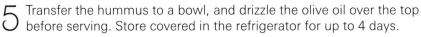

Calories **106** • Total fat **5g** • Saturated fat **1g** • Carbohydrate **10g** • Fiber **3g** • Protein **4g**

Creamy and spicy, with cool cucumber and garlic, this dip is delicious and addictive. It's great as a dip for vegetables or meats, but also as a spread for sandwiches.

TZATZIKI
(GREEK YOGURT AND GARLIC DIP)

 5 SERVINGS 7 MINUTES NONE 3 TABLESPOONS

1 medium English cucumber, peeled

2 garlic cloves, crushed

¼ tsp fine sea salt

Pinch of freshly ground black pepper

8oz (225g) full-fat Greek yogurt

2 tbsp plus 1 tsp extra virgin olive oil, divided

2 tbsp red wine vinegar

1 tbsp chopped fresh dill

1 Kalamata olive, pitted

1 In a medium bowl, grate the cucumber and then place it in the center of a tea towel. Pull the corners of the towel together and twist to squeeze as much water from the cucumber as possible. (This will prevent the dip from becoming watery.). Set aside.

2 In a small bowl, combine the garlic, sea salt, and black pepper. Mix until a paste is formed.

3 Add the Greek yogurt to a medium bowl. Whip the yogurt until it is creamy and then add the garlic paste. Mix well. Add the grated cucumber and mix again.

4 While continuously mixing, begin adding 2 tablespoons of the olive oil in small amounts, alternating with small amounts of the vinegar. When all of the olive oil and vinegar have been added, add the dill and mix well.

5 Drizzle the remaining 1 teaspoon of olive oil over the top, then garnish with the Kalamata olive. Cover the bowl with plastic wrap and transfer the dip to the refrigerator to rest for a minimum of 1 hour before serving. Store in the refrigerator for up to 4 days.

EACH SERVING HAS:

Calories **81** • Total fat **6g** • Saturated fat **2g** • Carbohydrate **3g** • Fiber **1g** • Protein **4g**

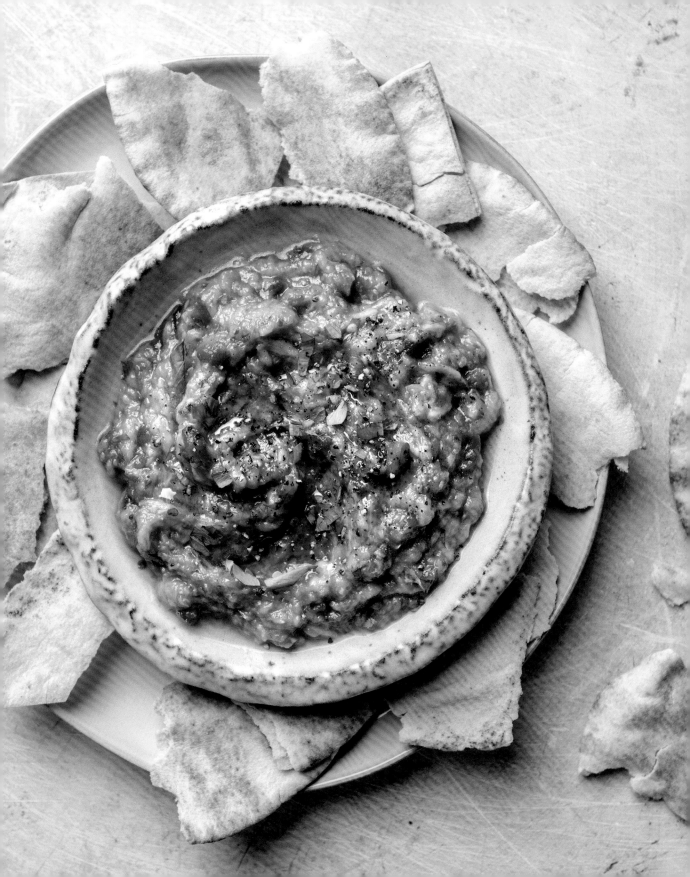

This rustic eggplant dip is chunky and flavorful—the garlic and vinegar complement the roasted eggplant to create a sweet and zesty dip. Serve as an appetizer with crunchy pita, fresh bread, or breadsticks.

EASY EGGPLANT DIP

 8 SERVINGS   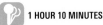 **1 HOUR 10 MINUTES**   **1 HOUR**   **3 TABLESPOONS**

1 medium globe eggplant (about 1lb/450g)

1 medium red bell pepper

1 large garlic clove, minced

½ tbsp red wine vinegar

¼ tbsp fine sea salt

2 tbsp finely chopped fresh parsley

1½ tbsp extra virgin olive oil

1 Preheat the oven to 400°F (200°C).

2 Use a fork to puncture the eggplant and bell pepper. Place them in a small roasting pan and roast for 1 hour or until both become soft, then remove the pan from the oven and set aside to cool for 5 minutes or until they're cool enough to handle.

3 Cut the cooled eggplant in half lengthwise and peel. (If peeling is difficult, use a spoon to scoop out the eggplant.) Transfer the eggplant to a food processor and pulse 3–4 times or until the texture becomes chunky, then transfer to a medium bowl. Seed and dice the bell pepper.

4 Add the bell pepper, garlic, vinegar, sea salt, and parsley to the bowl with the eggplant. Mix well, then gradually begin adding the olive oil, stirring continuously, until it's combined with the other ingredients.

5 Cover the dip with plastic wrap and transfer to the refrigerator to rest for a minimum of 1 hour before serving. Store in the refrigerator for up to 4 days.

EACH SERVING HAS:

Calories **68** • Total fat **4g** • Saturated fat **1g** • Carbohydrate **7g** • Fiber **4g** • Protein **1g**

This easy and flavorful Mediterranean-inspired dip is made with red peppers, feta cheese, Greek yogurt, and garlic. Serve as a dip with your favorite veggies or as a spread on bread or crackers. You can even use it as a sauce to accompany meat.

CHUNKY RED PEPPER AND FETA DIP

 5 SERVINGS   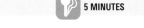 **5 MINUTES**   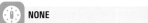 **NONE**   **3 TABLESPOONS**

2 jarred roasted red peppers

4 whole walnuts, shelled, divided

3 tbsp 2% Greek yogurt

1 tbsp extra virgin olive oil

¼ tsp dried oregano

¼ tsp freshly ground black pepper

1 garlic clove, quartered

1 tbsp unseasoned breadcrumbs

1.5oz (40g) crumbed feta

1 | Combine the red peppers, 3 walnuts, Greek yogurt, olive oil, oregano, black pepper, and garlic in a food processor. Process until the ingredients are chopped and blended. (The texture should be grainy.)

2 | Add the breadcrumbs to the mixture and stir. Add the feta and stir again.

3 | Transfer to a bowl and top with 1 chopped walnut. Store covered in the refrigerator for up to 2 days.

EACH SERVING HAS:

Calories **80** • Total fat **6g** • Saturated fat **2g** • Carbohydrate **3g** • Fiber **1g** • Protein **3g**

This spicy and tangy feta dip is perfectly creamy thanks to the Greek yogurt and olive oil. This is delicious as a dip, but even better as a spread on a sandwich or bruschetta.

TIROKAFTERI
(SPICY FETA AND YOGURT DIP)

8 SERVINGS	10 MINUTES	NONE	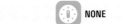 3 TABLESPOONS

1 tsp red wine vinegar

1 small green chili, seeded and sliced

2 tsp extra virgin olive oil

9oz (250g) full-fat feta

¾ cup full-fat Greek yogurt

1 Combine the vinegar, chili, and olive oil in a food processor. Blend until smooth.

2 In a small bowl, combine the feta and Greek yogurt, and use a fork to mash the ingredients until a paste is formed. Add the pepper mixture and stir until blended.

3 Cover and transfer to the refrigerator to chill for at least 1 hour before serving. Store covered in the refrigerator for up to 3 days.

 TIP

This can be served right away, but allowing it to chill in the refrigerator allows the flavors to meld.

EACH SERVING HAS:

Calories **167** • Total fat **13g** • Saturated fat **8g** • Carbohydrate **3g** • Fiber **0g** • Protein **9g**

These delicious figs are bite-sized energy snacks! Satisfying and filling, they're filled with nuts and topped with a touch of honey. Enjoy them as is, or serve over a bowl of yogurt for a light meal.

ROASTED STUFFED FIGS

 5 SERVINGS   **5 MINUTES**   **10 MINUTES**   **2 FIGS**

10 medium dried figs

1½ tbsp finely chopped walnuts

1½ tbsp finely chopped almonds

½ tsp ground cinnamon

½ tsp sesame seeds

Pinch of salt

1½ tsp honey

1 Preheat the oven to 300°F (150°C). Line a large baking sheet with foil, and grease the foil with olive oil.

2 Using a sharp knife, make a small vertical cut into the side of each fig, making sure not to cut all the way through the fig. Set aside.

3 In a small bowl, combine the walnuts, almonds, cinnamon, sesame seeds, and salt. Mix well.

4 Stuff each fig with 1 teaspoon of the filling, gently pressing the filling into the figs. Place the figs on the prepared baking sheet, and bake for 10 minutes.

5 While the figs are baking, add the honey to a small saucepan over medium heat. Heat the honey for 30 seconds or until it becomes thin and watery.

6 Transfer the roasted figs to a plate. Drizzle a few drops of the warm honey over each fig before serving. Store in an airtight container in the refrigerator for up to 2 weeks.

EACH SERVING HAS:

Calories **80** • Total fat **3g** • Saturated fat **1g** • Carbohydrate **13g** • Fiber **2g** • Protein **1g**

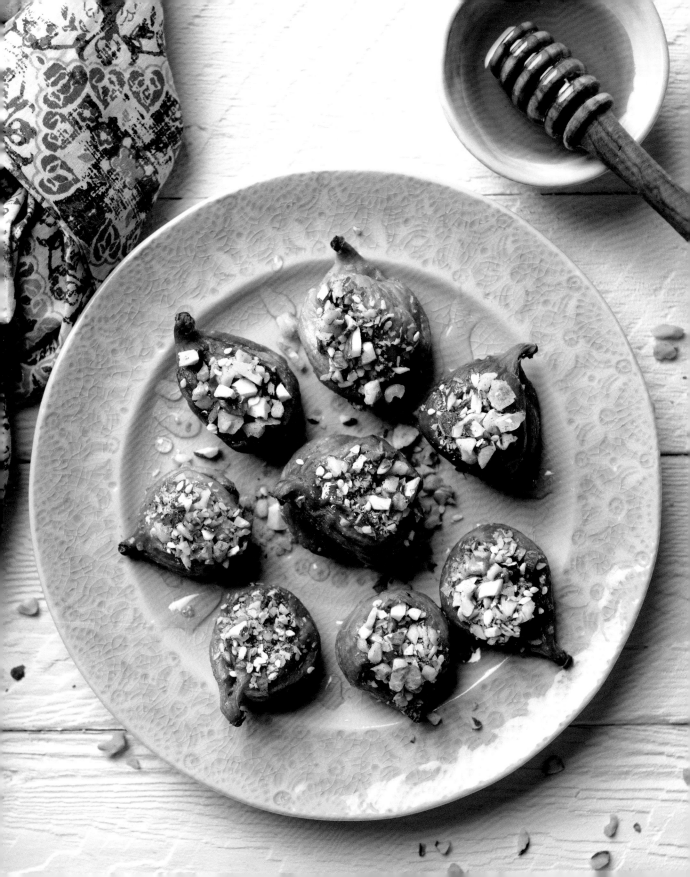

Crispy cucumber slices are topped with a light and creamy tuna salad made with tangy Greek yogurt. Seasoned with fresh dill and spring onion, this is a light and filling snack.

NO-MAYO TUNA SALAD CUCUMBER BITES

 3 SERVINGS **5 MINUTES** **NONE** **5 BITES**

1 (5oz/140g) can water-packed tuna, drained

⅓ cup full-fat Greek yogurt

½ tsp extra virgin olive oil

1 tbsp finely chopped spring onion (white parts only)

1 tbsp chopped fresh dill

Pinch of coarse sea salt

¼ tsp freshly ground black pepper

1 medium cucumber, cut into 15 (¼-inch/.5cm) thick slices

1 tsp red wine vinegar

1 In a medium bowl, combine the tuna, yogurt, olive oil, spring onion, dill, sea salt, and black pepper. Mix well.

2 Arrange the cucumber slices on a plate and sprinkle the vinegar over the slices.

3 Place 1 heaping teaspoon of the tuna salad on top of each cucumber slice

4 Serve promptly. Store the tuna salad mixture covered in the refrigerator for up to 1 day.

EACH SERVING HAS:

Calories **109** • Total fat **4g** • Saturated fat **1g** • Carbohydrate **5g** • Fiber **1g** • Protein **14g**

This light and savory snack features the classic Greek combination of spinach and feta. It's a quick and convenient recipe that is a perfect snack for any time of the day.

MEDITERRANEAN MINI SPINACH QUICHE

 5 SERVINGS   15 MINUTES   25 MINUTES   2 MINI QUICHE

2 tsp extra virgin olive oil plus extra for greasing pan

3 eggs

3oz (85g) crumbled feta

4 tbsp grated Parmesan cheese, divided

¼ tsp freshly ground black pepper

6oz (170g) frozen spinach, thawed and chopped

1 tbsp chopped fresh mint

1 tbsp chopped fresh dill

1 Preheat the oven to 375°F (190°C). Liberally grease a 10-cup muffin pan with olive oil.

2 In a medium bowl, combine the eggs, feta, 3 tablespoons of the Parmesan, black pepper, and 2 teaspoons of the olive oil. Mix well. Add the spinach, mint, and dill, and mix to combine.

3 Fill each muffin cup with 1 heaping tablespoon of the batter. Sprinkle the remaining Parmesan over the quiche.

4 Bake for 25 minutes or until the egg is set and the tops are golden. Set aside to cool for 3 minutes, then remove the quiche from the pan by running a knife around the edges of each muffin cup. Transfer the quiche to a wire rack to cool completely.

5 Store in the refrigerator for up to 3 days or freeze for up to 3 months. (If freezing, individually wrap each quiche in plastic wrap and then in foil.)

 TIP
Make sure the muffin cups are well greased to ensure the quiche don't stick to the pan. You can also use a silicone muffin pan.

EACH SERVING HAS:

Calories **141** • Total fat **10g** • Saturated fat **5g** • Carbohydrate **3g** • Fiber **1g** • Protein **9g**

CHAPTER EIGHT
DESSERTS

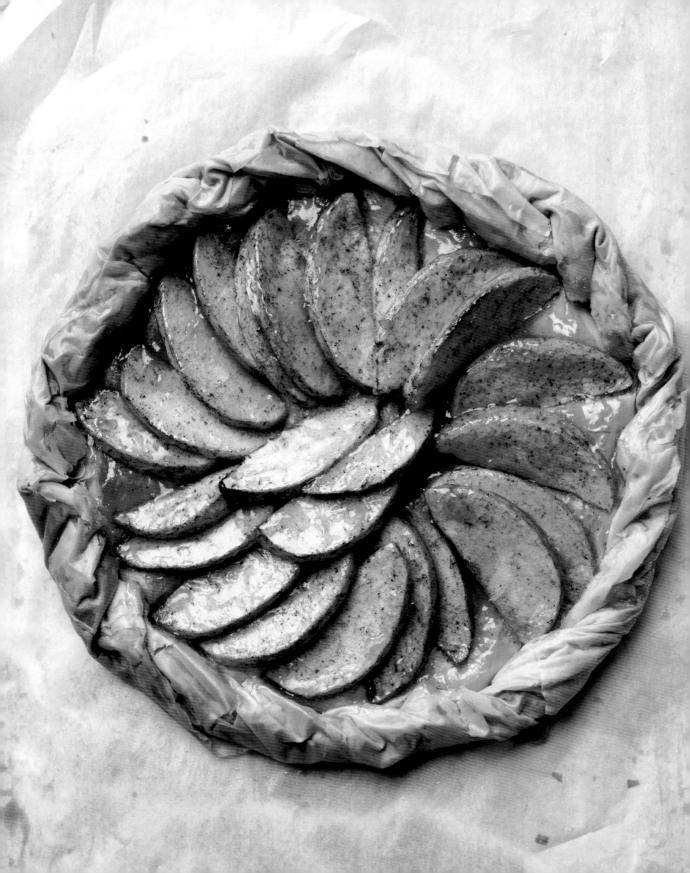

Satisfy your sweet tooth with a light tart of roasted apples nestled in crispy phyllo dough. Enjoy this treat warm or at room temperature, served with a dollop of Greek yogurt.

CRISPY APPLE PHYLLO TART

 4 SERVINGS   **15 MINUTES**   **30 MINUTES**   **¼ TART**

5 tsp extra virgin olive oil

2 tsp fresh lemon juice

¼ tsp ground cinnamon

1½ tsp granulated sugar, divided

1 large apple (any variety), peeled and cut into ⅛-inch (3mm) thick slices

5 (14 x 18-in/35.5 x 46cm) phyllo sheets, defrosted

1 tsp all-purpose flour

1½ tsp apricot jam

1 Preheat the oven to 350°F (180°C). Line a baking sheet with parchment paper, and pour the olive oil into a small dish. Set aside.

2 In a separate small bowl, combine the lemon juice, cinnamon, 1 teaspoon of the sugar, and the apple slices. Mix well to ensure the apple slices are coated in the seasonings. Set aside.

3 On a clean working surface, stack the phyllo sheets one on top of the other. Place a large bowl with an approximate diameter of 15 inches (38cm) on top of the sheets, then draw a sharp knife around the edge of the bowl to cut out a circle through all 5 sheets. Discard the remaining phyllo.

4 Working quickly, place the first sheet on the lined baking sheet and then brush with the olive oil. Repeat the process by placing a second sheet on top of the first sheet, then brushing the second sheet with olive oil. Repeat until all the phyllo sheets are in a single stack.

5 Sprinkle the flour and remaining sugar over the top of the sheets. Arrange the apples in overlapping circles 4 inches (10cm) from the edge of the phyllo.

6 Fold the edges of the phyllo in and then twist them all around the apple filling to form a crust edge. Brush the edge with the remaining olive oil. Bake for 30 minutes or until the crust is golden and the apples are browned on the edges.

7 While the tart is baking, heat the apricot jam in a small sauce pan over low heat until it's melted.

8 When the tart is done baking, brush the apples with the jam sauce. Slice the tart into 4 equal servings and serve warm. Store at room temperature, covered in plastic wrap, for up to 2 days.

EACH SERVING HAS:

Calories **259** • Total fat **18g** • Saturated fat **3g** • Carbohydrate **23g** • Fiber **2g** • Protein **2g**

Ground walnuts, cinnamon, and olive oil give this rich cake its characteristic nutty and deep flavor. It's finished with a light syrup for a decadent but healthy treat.

KARITHOPITA
(GREEK JUICY WALNUT CAKE)

 8 SERVINGS   10 MINUTES   🕐 30 MINUTES   🍴 1 SLICE

¼ cup extra virgin olive oil plus 1 tsp for brushing

½ cup walnut halves

¼ cup granulated sugar

¼ cup brown sugar

1 egg

1 tbsp pure vanilla extract

¼ cup orange juice, strained

½ cup all-purpose flour

¼ cup whole-wheat flour

¼ tsp baking powder

¼ tsp baking soda

¼ tsp ground cinnamon

For the syrup

⅓ cup water

¼ cup granulated sugar

1 cinnamon stick

1 tbsp orange juice

1 Preheat the oven to 350°F (180°C). Brush an 8 × 4-inch (20 × 10cm) loaf pan with 1 teaspoon of the olive oil, and then line the pan with parchment paper.

2 Prepare the syrup by combining the water, sugar, and cinnamon stick in a small pan placed over medium heat. Bring to a boil and then boil for 2 minutes, then remove the pan from the heat. Remove the cinnamon stick, add the orange juice, then stir and set aside to cool.

3 Pulse the walnuts in a food processor until you achieve a cornmeal-like consistency. (Do not over-grind.)

4 In a large bowl, combine ¼ cup of the olive oil, the granulated sugar, and the brown sugar. Stir until the sugar is dissolved, then add the egg. Add the vanilla extract and orange juice. Mix well.

5 In a small bowl, combine the all-purpose flour and whole-wheat flour with the baking powder, baking soda, and cinnamon.

6 Add the flour mixture to the olive oil mixture and mix just until the flour has been incorporated. Add ¼ cup of the ground walnuts and mix until they are distributed throughout the batter.

7 Pour the batter into the prepared pan. Bake for 25–30 minutes or until a toothpick inserted into the cake comes out clean.

8 Use a toothpick to poke 8 holes across the top of the cake and then pour the syrup over the entire surface of the cake. Sprinkle the remaining ground walnuts over the top, and then set the cake aside to rest for 30 minutes before cutting it in equal-sized 1-inch slices. Store in an airtight container in the refrigerator for up to 5 days.

EACH SERVING HAS:

Calories **239** • Total fat **13g** • Saturated fat **2g** • Carbohydrate **28g** • Fiber **1g** • Protein **3g**

Inspired by a traditional Greek olive oil and yogurt cake recipe, these light and moist, lemon-flavored cupcakes have a touch of tanginess.

LIGHT AND LEMONY OLIVE OIL CUPCAKES

 18 SERVINGS   **10 MINUTES**   **22–25 MINUTES**   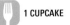 **1 CUPCAKE**

2 cups all-purpose flour

4 tsp baking powder

1 cup granulated sugar

1 cup extra virgin olive oil

2 eggs

7oz (200g) 2% Greek yogurt

1 tsp pure vanilla extract

4 tbsp fresh lemon juice

Zest of 2 lemons

For the glaze

1 tbsp lemon juice

5 tbsp powdered sugar

1 Preheat the oven to 350°F (180°C). Line a 12-cup muffin pan with cupcake liners and then line a second pan with 6 liners. Set aside.

2 In a medium bowl, combine the flour and baking powder. Whisk and set aside.

3 In a large bowl, combine the sugar and olive oil, and mix until smooth. Add the eggs, one at a time, and mix well. Add the Greek yogurt, vanilla extract, lemon juice, and lemon zest. Mix until well combined.

4 Add the flour mixture to the batter, ½ cup at a time, while continuously mixing.

5 Spoon the batter into the liners, filling each liner two-thirds full. Bake for 22–25 minutes or until a toothpick inserted into the center of a cupcake comes out clean.

6 While the cupcakes are baking, make the glaze by combining the lemon juice and powdered sugar in a small bowl. Stir until smooth, then set aside.

7 Set the cupcakes aside to cool in the pans for about 5 minutes, then remove the cupcakes from the pans and transfer to a wire rack to cool completely.

8 Drizzle the glaze over the cooled cupcakes. Store in the refrigerator for up to 4 days.

EACH SERVING HAS:

Calories **227**   •   Total fat **13g**   •   Saturated fat **2g**   •   Carbohydrate **25g**   •   Fiber **1g**   •   Protein **3g**

These traditional crunchy, cinnamon-flavored cookies are made with olive oil, sugar, and flour—no eggs, butter, or milk. They're perfect for dipping in coffee, tea, or milk.

KOULOURAKIA
(OLIVE OIL CINNAMON COOKIES)

15 SERVINGS · **25 MINUTES** · **25–30 MINUTES** · **2 COOKIES**

¼ cup extra virgin olive oil

¼ cup granulated sugar

¼ cup orange juice, strained

1¼ cups all-purpose flour plus extra if needed

¼ tsp baking powder

¼ tsp baking soda

¼ tsp ground cinnamon

For the cinnamon-sugar coating

1½ tbsp granulated sugar

¾ tsp ground cinnamon

1 Preheat the oven to 350°F (180°C). Line a large baking sheet with parchment paper.

2 In a large bowl, combine the olive oil, sugar, and orange juice. Mix with a rubber spatula until the sugar has completely dissolved.

3 In a small bowl, combine the flour, baking powder, baking soda, and cinnamon. Stir to combine.

4 Gradually add the flour mixture to the olive oil mixture while gently mixing and folding with the spatula until a smooth, shiny, pliable dough that does not stick to your hands is formed. Pick up the dough with your hands and fold it once or twice to make sure it has the proper consistency. If the dough is still sticky, add more flour in small amounts. (Be careful not to add more flour than needed.) Cover the dough with plastic wrap and set it aside to rest for 5 minutes at room temperature.

5 While the dough is resting, make the cinnamon-sugar coating by combining the sugar and cinnamon in a small bowl and mixing well.

6 When the dough is rested, coat your fingers with a few drops of olive oil and begin shaping the cookies by taking about 1 teaspoon of the dough and rolling it out into a thin cord about 6 inches long, then set it aside. Continue the process until you have 10–12 cords, then dip each cord in the cinnamon-sugar mixture and fold it in half and twist it into a braid, or shape it into a ring or spiral. Place the cookies on the prepared baking sheet, and bake for 12–15 minutes or until golden brown.

7 While the first batch is baking, begin shaping the next batch. Once the first batch is done baking, remove the pan from the oven and let them sit for 5 minutes before transferring them to a wire rack to cool completely. Repeat the process with the remaining dough. Store in an airtight container for up to 3 weeks.

EACH SERVING HAS:

Calories **89** · Total fat **4g** · Saturated fat **1g** · Carbohydrate **13g** · Fiber **0g** · Protein **1g**

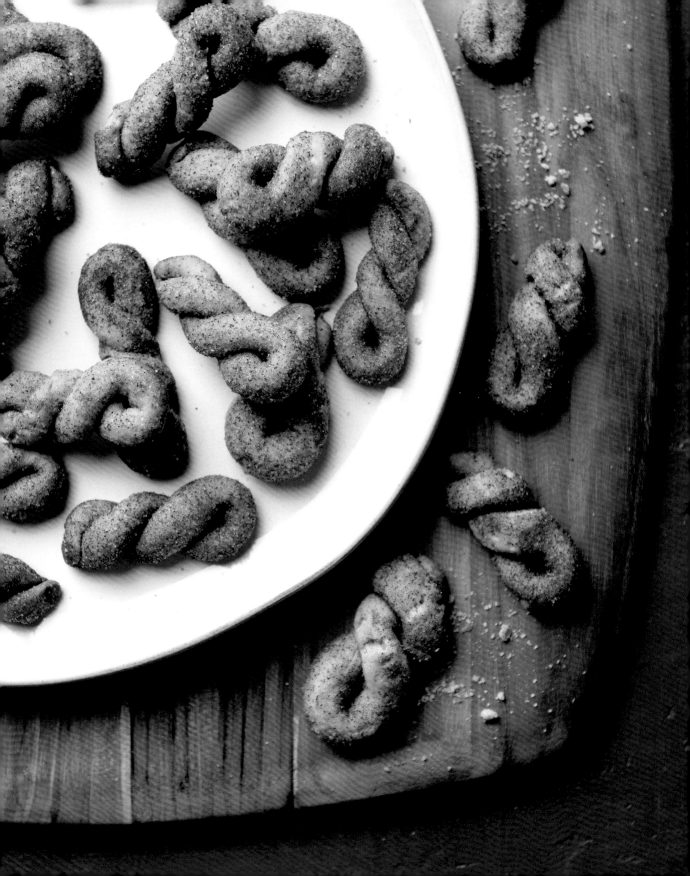

These lightened-up brownies are moist and full of rich chocolate flavor. The olive oil adds another dimension of flavor to this popular Mediterranean dessert. These are easy to make, and in no time at all you'll have a nice chocolate dessert to share with guests.

OLIVE OIL GREEK YOGURT BROWNIES

 9 SERVINGS   5 MINUTES   25 MINUTES   1 BROWNIE

¼ cup extra virgin olive oil

¾ cup granulated sugar

1 tsp pure vanilla extract

2 eggs

¼ cup 2% Greek yogurt

½ cup all-purpose flour

⅓ cup unsweetened cocoa powder

¼ tsp salt

¼ tsp baking powder

⅓ cup chopped walnuts

1 Preheat the oven to 350°F (180°C) and line a 9-inch (22cm) square baking pan with wax paper.

2 In a small bowl, combine the olive oil and sugar. Stir until well combined, then add the vanilla extract and mix well.

3 In another small bowl, beat the eggs and then add them to the olive oil mixture. Mix well. Add the yogurt and mix again.

4 In medium bowl, combine the flour, cocoa powder, salt, and baking powder, then mix well. Add the olive oil mixture to the dry ingredients and mix well, then add the walnuts and mix again.

5 Carefully pour the brownie mixture into the prepared pan and use a spatula to smooth the top. Transfer to the oven and bake for 25 minutes.

6 Set the brownies aside to cool completely. Lift the wax paper to remove the brownies from the pan. Remove the paper and cut the brownies into 9 squares. Store at room temperature in an airtight container for up to 2 days.

 TIP

Make sure you use the right size pan; otherwise the brownies will be very thin and may become overcooked and dry.

EACH SERVING HAS:

Calories **207** • Total fat **10g** • Saturated fat **2g** • Carbohydrate **25g** • Fiber **2g** • Protein **4g**

This delicious mousse is creamy, rich, and refreshing. The combination of tangy yogurt and sweet ricotta has the flavor of cheesecake, but without all the calories. Drizzle with a bit of strawberry or cherry syrup for extra flavor.

GREEK YOGURT RICOTTA MOUSSE

 4 SERVINGS   **1 HOUR 5 MINUTES**   ⏲ **NONE**   🍴 **½ CUP**

9oz (250g) full-fat ricotta cheese

4.5oz (125g) 2% Greek yogurt

3 tsp fresh lemon juice

½ tsp pure vanilla extract

2 tbsp granulated sugar

1 | Combine all of the ingredients in a food processor. Blend until smooth, about 1 minute.

2 | Divide the mousse between 4 serving glasses. Cover and transfer to the refrigerator to chill for 1 hour before serving. Store covered in the refrigerator for up to 4 days.

TIP
This is delicious served as is, or topped with fresh seasonal fruit.

EACH SERVING HAS:
Calories **159** • Total fat **9g** • Saturated fat **6g** • Carbohydrate **10g** • Fiber **0g** • Protein **10g**

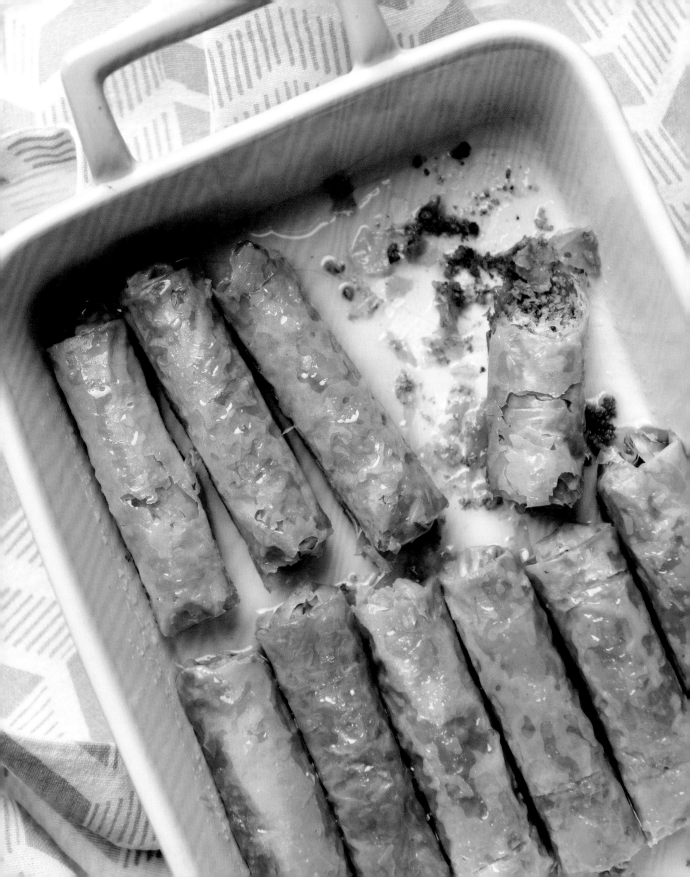

Flaky, crunchy phyllo dough is wrapped around a sweet walnut and cinnamon filling and drenched with a lemon-flavored syrup in this favorite Mediterranean treat.

LIGHTENED-UP BAKLAVA ROLLS
(WALNUT PHYLLO ROLLS)

 12 SERVINGS   **2 MINUTES** **1 HOUR 15 MINUTES**   **1 ROLL**

4oz (115g) shelled walnuts

1¼ tsp ground cinnamon

1½ tsp granulated sugar

5 tsp unseasoned breadcrumbs

1 tsp extra virgin olive oil plus 2 tbsp for brushing

6 (14 x 18-in/35.5 x 46cm) phyllo sheets, defrosted

For the syrup:

¼ cup water

½ cup granulated sugar

1½ tbsp fresh lemon juice

1 Preheat the oven to 350°F (180°C).

2 Make the syrup by combining the water and sugar in a small pan placed over medium heat. Bring to a boil, cook for 2 minutes, then remove the pan from the heat. Add the lemon juice, and stir. Set aside to cool.

3 In a food processor, combine the walnuts, cinnamon, sugar, breadcrumbs, and 1 teaspoon of the olive oil. Pulse until combined and grainy, but not chunky.

4 Place 1 phyllo sheet on a clean working surface and brush with the olive oil. Place a second sheet on top of the first sheet, brush with olive oil, and repeat the process with a third sheet. Cut the sheets in half crosswise, and then cut each half into 3 pieces crosswise.

5 Scatter 1 tablespoon of the walnut mixture over the phyllo sheet. Start rolling the phyllo and filling into a log shape while simultaneously folding the sides in (like a burrito) until the filling is encased in each piece of dough. The rolls should be about 3½ inches long. Place the rolls one next to the other in a large baking pan, then repeat the process with the remaining 3 phyllo sheets. You should have a total of 12 rolls.

6 Lightly brush the rolls with the remaining olive oil. Place in the oven to bake for 30 minutes or until the rolls turn golden brown, then remove from the oven and promptly drizzle the cold syrup over the top.

7 Let the rolls sit for 20 minutes, then flip them over and let them sit for an additional 20 minutes. Turn them over once more and sprinkle any remining walnut mixture over the rolls before serving. Store uncovered at room temperature for 2 days (to retain crispiness) and then cover with plastic wrap and store at room temperature for up to 10 days.

EACH SERVING HAS:

Calories **133** • Total fat **9g** • Saturated fat **1g** • Carbohydrate **12g** • Fiber **1g** • Protein **8g**

The original energy bites! These nutty sweets are made the traditional way, with ground roasted almonds, a bit of sugar, and cocoa.

GREEK ISLAND
ALMOND COCOA BiTES

 6 SERVINGS   **5 MINUTES**   🕐 **NONE**   🍴 **2 BITES**

½ cup roasted, unsalted whole almonds (with skins)

3 tbsp granulated sugar, divided

1½ tsp unsweetened cocoa powder

1¼ tbsp unseasoned breadcrumbs

¾ tsp pure vanilla extract

1½ tsp orange juice

1 Place the almonds in a food processor and process until you have a coarse ground texture.

2 In a medium bowl, combine the ground almonds, 2 tablespoons sugar, the cocoa powder, and the breadcrumbs. Mix well.

3 In a small bowl, combine the vanilla extract and orange juice. Stir and then add the mixture to the almond mixture. Mix well.

4 Measure out a teaspoon of the mixture. Squeeze the mixture with your hand to make the dough stick together, then mold the dough into a small ball.

5 Add the remaining tablespoon of the sugar to a shallow bowl. Roll the balls in the sugar until covered, then transfer the bites to an airtight container. Store covered at room temperature for up to 1 week.

 TIP

If desired, you can substitute an equal amount of brandy for the vanilla extract.

EACH SERVING HAS:

Calories **104** • Total fat **6g** • Saturated fat **1g** • Carbohydrate **10g** • Fiber **1g** • Protein **3g**

Dried apricots are poached in an aromatic syrup until tender, paired with pistachios, and served with a creamy Greek yogurt and mascarpone blend in this delightful dessert.

POACHED APRICOTS AND PISTACHIOS
WITH GREEK YOGURT

 4 SERVINGS   2 MINUTES   18 MINUTES   3 APRICOTS

½ cup orange juice

2 tbsp brandy

2 tbsp honey

¾ cup water

1 cinnamon stick

12 dried apricots

⅓ cup 2% Greek yogurt

2 tbsp mascarpone cheese

2 tbsp shelled pistachios

1 Place a saucepan over medium heat and add the orange juice, brandy, honey, and water. Stir to combine, then add the cinnamon stick.

2 Once the honey has dissolved, add the apricots. Bring the mixture to a boil, then cover, reduce the heat to low, and simmer for 15 minutes.

3 While the apricots are simmering, combine the Greek yogurt and mascarpone cheese in a small serving bowl. Stir until smooth, then set aside.

4 When the cooking time for the apricots is complete, uncover, add the pistachios, and continue simmering for 3 more minutes. Remove the pan from the heat.

5 To serve, divide the Greek yogurt–mascarpone cheese mixture into 4 serving bowls and top each serving with 3 apricots, a few pistachios, and 1 teaspoon of the syrup. The apricots and syrup can be stored in a jar at room temperature for up to 1 month.

 TIP

These apricots also are delicious served over cereal, in oatmeal, over pancakes or waffles, or even enjoyed on their own.

EACH SERVING HAS:

Calories **195**   •   Total fat **8g**   •   Saturated fat **5g**   •   Carbohydrate **27g**   •   Fiber **2g**   •   Protein **4g**

REFERENCES

Ajala O., English P., Pinkney J. Systematic Review and Meta-analysis of Different Dietary Approaches to the Management of Type 2 Diabetes. *Am. J. Clin. Nutr.* 2013; 97(3): 505–516.

Allbaugh L. Crete: A Case Study of an Underdeveloped Area. Princeton, NJ. Princeton University Press; 1953.

Allouche Y., Jiménez A., Gaforio J.J., Uceda M., Beltrán G. How Heating Affects Extra Virgin Olive Oil Quality Indexes and Chemical Composition. *J. Agric. Food Chem.* 2007; 55 (23): 9646–9654.

Anastasiou C.A., Yannakoulia M., Kosmidis M.H., et al. Mediterranean Diet and Cognitive Health: Initial Results From the Hellenic Longitudinal Investigation of Ageing and Diet. *PLoS One.* 2017; 12(8): e0182048.

Argyropoulos K., et al. Adherence to Mediterranean Diet and Risk of Late-Life Depression. Presented at: APA Annual Meeting; May 18–22, 2019; San Francisco.

Benetou, V., Orfanos, P., Pettersson-Kymmer, U. et al. Mediterranean Diet and Incidence of Hip Fractures in a European Cohort. *Osteoporosis Int.* 24, 2013; 1587–1598.

Beunza J.J., Toledo E., Hu F.B., et al. Adherence to the Mediterranean Diet, Long-Term Weight Change and Incident Overweight or Obesity: The Seguimiento Universidad de Navarra (SUN) cohort. *Am. J. Clin. Nutr.* 2010; 92 (6): 1484–1493.

Boghossian N.S., Yeung E.H., Mumford S.L., et al. Adherence to the Mediterranean Diet and Body Fat Distribution in Reproductive Aged Women. *Eur. J. Clin. Nutr.* 2013; 67 (3): 289–294.

Cao M., Li D., Li K., et al. An Epidemiological Study on the Relationship Between the Siesta and Blood Pressure. *National Medical Journal of China*. 2016; 96 (21), 1699–1701.

Dehghan M., Mente A., Zhang X., et al. Associations of Fats and Carbohydrate Intake with Cardiovascular Disease and Mortality in 18 Countries From Five Continents (PURE): A Prospective Cohort Study. *Lancet.* 2017; 390 (10107): 2050–2062.

Estruch R., Ros E., Salas-Salvadó J., et al. Retraction and Republication: Primary Prevention of Cardiovascular Disease with a Mediterranean Diet. *N. Engl. J. Med.* 2013; 368: 1279–90 [retraction of: *N. Engl. J. Med.* 2013 Apr 4; 368 (14): 1279–90]. *N. Engl. J. Med.* 2018; 378 (25): 2441–2442.

Féart C., Samieri C., Rondeau V., et al. Adherence to a Mediterranean Diet, Cognitive Decline and Risk of Dementia. *JAMA.* 2009; 302 (6): 638–648.

Fung T.T., Rexrode K.M., Mantzoros C.S., Manson J.E., Willett W.C., Hu F.B. Mediterranean Diet and Incidence of, and Mortality from, Coronary Heart Disease and Stroke in Women. Circulation. 2009; 119 (8): 1093–1100.

Galvão Cândido F., Xavier Valente F., da Silva L.E., et al. Consumption of Extra Virgin Olive Oil Improves Body Composition and Blood Pressure in Women with Excess Body Fat: A Randomized, Double-Blinded, Placebo-Controlled Clinical Trial. *Eur. J. Nutr.* 2018; 57 (7): 2445–2455.

Garcia-Martinez O., Ruiz C., Gutierrez-Ibanez A., Illescas-Montes R., Melguizo-Rodriguez L. Benefits of Olive Oil Phenolic Compounds in Disease Prevention. *Endocr. Metab. Immune Disord. Drug Targets.* 2018; 18 (4): 333–340.

Gibney M.J. Ultra-Processed Foods: Definitions and Policy Issues. *Curr. Dev. Nutr.* 2019; 3: 1–7.

Guillaume C., et al. Evaluation of Chemical and Physical Changes in Different Commercial Oils During Heating. *Acta Scientific Nutritional Health*, 2018; 2.6, 02–11.

Jacka F.N., O'Neil A., Opie R., et al. A Randomised Controlled Trial of Dietary Improvement for Adults with Major Depression (the SMILES Trial). *BMC Medicine* 2017; 15 (1): 23.

Keys A., Aravanis C., Blackburn H., Buzina, et al. Seven Countries. A Multivariate Analysis of Death and Coronary Heart Disease. Cambridge, MA and London: Harvard University Press. 1980.

Khaw K.T., Wareham N., Bingham S., Welch A., Luben R., Day N. Combined Impact of Health Behaviours and Mortality in Men and Women: the EPIC-Norfolk Prospective Population Study. *PLoS Medicine*. 2008; 5 (1): e12.

Kulovitz M.G., Kravitz L.R., Mermier C., et al. Potential Role of Meal Frequency as a Strategy for Weight Loss and Health in Overweight or Obese Adults. *Nutrition*. 2014; 30 (4): 386–392.

Lassale, C., Batty, G.D., Baghdadli, A. et al. Healthy Dietary Indices and Risk of Depressive Outcomes: A Systematic Review and Meta-analysis of Observational Studies. *Mol Psychiatry* 24, 2019; 965–986.

Lopez-Garcia E., Rodriguez-Artalejo F., Li T.Y., et al. The Mediterranean-Style Dietary Pattern and Mortality Among Men and Women with Cardiovascular Disease. *Am J Clin Nutr*. 2014; 99 (1): 172–180.

Mancini, J. G., Filion, K. B., Atallah, R., & Eisenberg, M. J. Systematic Review of the Mediterranean Diet for Long-Term Weight Loss. *The American Journal of Medicine*, 129 (4), 2016; 407–415.e4.

Martínez-González M.A., Gea A., Ruiz-Canela M. The Mediterranean Diet and Cardiovascular Health. *Circ Res*. 2019; 124 (5): 779–798.

Martínez-González M.A., de la Fuente-Arrillaga C., Nunez-Cordoba J.M., et al. Adherence to Mediterranean Diet and Risk of Developing Diabetes: Prospective Cohort Study. *BMJ*. 2008; 336 (7657): 1348–1351.

Nestle M. Mediterranean Diets: Historical and Research Overview. *Am. J. Clin. Nutr.* 1995; 61 (6 Suppl.): 1313S–1320S.

Panagiotakos D.B., Pitsavos C., Polychronopoulos E., Chrysohoou C., Zampelas A., Trichopoulou A. Can a Mediterranean Diet Moderate the Development and Clinical Progression of Coronary Heart Disease? A Systematic Review. *Med Sci Monit*. 2004; 10 (8): RA193–RA198.

Shai I., Schwarzfuchs D., Henkin Y., et al. (2009). Weight Loss With a Low-Carbohydrate, Mediterranean or Low-Fat Diet. *N. Engl. J. Med.* 2008; 359 (3): 229–241.

Schwingshackl, L., & Hoffmann, G. Adherence to Mediterranean Diet and Risk of Cancer: A Systematic Review and Meta-analysis of Observational Studies. *International Journal of Cancer*, 2014; 135 (8), 1884–1897.

Talegawkar S.A., Bandinelli S., Bandeen-Roche K., et al. A Higher Adherence to a Mediterranean-Style Diet is Inversely Associated with the Development of Frailty in Community-Dwelling Elderly Men and Women. *J. Nutr.* 2012; 142 (12): 2161–2166.

Toledo E, Salas-Salvadó J., Donat-Vargas C., et al. Mediterranean Diet and Invasive Breast Cancer Risk Among Women at High Cardiovascular Risk in the PREDIMED Trial: A Randomized Clinical Trial. *JAMA Intern. Med.* 2015; 175 (11): 1752–1760.

Trichopoulou A., Bamia C., Trichopoulos D. Mediterranean Diet and Survival Among Patients with Coronary Heart Disease in Greece. *Arch. Intern. Med.* 2005; 165 (8): 929–935.

Trichopoulou A., Vasilopoulou E., Georga K. Macro- and Micronutrients in a Traditional Greek Menu. *Forum Nutr.* 2005; (57): 135–146.

Waterman E., Lockwood B. Active Components and Clinical Applications of Olive Oil. *Altern. Med. Rev.* 2007; 12 (4): 331–342.

Willett W.C., Sacks F., Trichopoulou A., et al. Mediterranean Diet Pyramid: A Cultural Model for Healthy Eating. *Am. J. Clin. Nutr.* 1995; 61 (6 Suppl): 1402S–1406S.

INDEX

A

alcohol consumption, 19

appetizers

Baked Italian Spinach and Ricotta Balls, 156–157

Chunky Red Pepper and Feta Dip, 166

Classic Hummus, 162

Easy Eggplant Dip, 164–165

Kalamata Olive Tapenade, 154

Loaded Vegetable Pita Pizzas with Tahini Sauce, 158

Mediterranean Mini Spinach Quiche, 171

Mediterranean Lentil Bowl, 159

No-Mayo Tuna Salad Cucumber Bites, 170

Roasted Stuffed Figs, 168–169

Sardine and Herb Bruschetta, 152–153

Stuffed Dates with Feta, Parmesan, and Pine Nuts, 160–161

Mediterranean-Style Stuffed Mushrooms, 155

Tirokafteri (Spicy Feta and Yogurt Dip), 167

Tzatziki (Greek Yogurt and Garlic Dip), 163

Arugula Spinach Salad with Shaved Parmesan, 144

B

Baked Italian Spinach and Ricotta Balls, 156–157

beans, 22, 55

selecting, 24

beef, 17

Bifteki (Mediterranean Burgers), 121

Hearty Stewed Beef in Tomato Sauce, 117

Spiced Oven-Baked Meatballs with Tomato Sauce, 120

Beet and Walnut Salad, 134–135

beverages, 16, 23

Bifteki (Mediterranean Burgers), 121

brain health, 15

Braised Cauliflower, 70–71

braising, 28

bread, 23

breakfasts, 21, 30

Bulgur Wheat Cereal with Apples and Almonds, 41

Greek Yogurt Breakfast Bowl with Almonds, Banana, and Tahini, 38–39

Kagianas (Scrambled Eggs with Feta and Tomato), 50

Mediterranean Breakfast Pita Sandwiches, 48–49

Mediterranean Omelet, 40

Mediterranean-Inspired White Smoothie, 51

Ricotta and Fruit Bruschetta, 42–43

Savory Feta, Spinach, and Red Pepper Muffins, 44

Savory Zucchini Muffins, 45

Shakshuka (Poached Egg on Tomatoes with Spices and Onion), 46–47

Tiropita (Greek Cheese Pie), 52–53

Briami (Sheet Pan Roasted Vegetables), 74–75

bulgur wheat, 41

Bulgur Wheat Cereal with Apples and Almonds, 41

C

Cabbage and Carrot Salad, 137

cancer prevention, 14

canned beans, 29

canned tomatoes, 29

Caponata (Sicilian Eggplant), 56–57

carbohydrates, 17

casserole dishes, 52

Chicken Souvlaki, 113

Chickpea Patties with Tomato Sauce, 73

Chickpeas with Spinach and Sun-Dried Tomatoes, 76

child-friendly substitutions, 19

Chunky Red Pepper and Feta Dip, 166

Citrus Avocado Salad, 148

Citrus Mediterranean Salmon with Lemon Caper Sauce, 106–107

Classic Hummus, 162

Classic Tabbouleh, 129

coffee, 21

Cretan Roasted Zucchini, 62–63

Crispy Apple Phyllo Tart, 174–175

Crustless Savory Zucchini and Feta Pie, 89

D

dairy products, 16, 23

selecting, 25

Dakos (Cretan Salad), 138–139

desserts, 16, 23

Crispy Apple Phyllo Tart, 174–175

Greek Island Almond Cocoa Bites, 184

Greek Yogurt Ricotta Mousse, 181